Pre-Exercise Health Screening Guide

Tim Olds, PhD, and Kevin Norton, PhD
University of South Australia

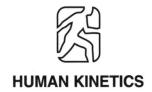

HUMAN KINETICS

Library of Congress Cataloging-in-Publication Data

Olds, Tim.
    Pre-exercise health screening guide / Timothy Olds and Kevin
Norton.
      p. cm.
    Includes bibliographical references.
    ISBN 0-7360-0210-3
    1. Athletes--Medical examinations.   2. Physical fitness.
I. Norton, Kevin.   II. Title.
RC1225.043   1999
613.7'088'796--dc21   99-24274
                                    CIP

ISBN: 0-7360-0210-3

Developmental Editor: Joyce Atkinson
Copyeditor: Andrew Smith
Proofreader: Erin Cler
Graphic Designer: Stuart Cartwright
Cover Designer: Keith Blomberg
Illustrator: Chuck Nivens
Printer: Versa

Printed in the United States of America

10   9   8   7   6   5   4   3   2   1

HumanKinetics
Web site: http://www.humankinetics.com/

United States: Human Kinetics, P.O. Box 5076, Champaign, IL 61825-5076
1-800-747-4457
e-mail: humank@hkusa.com

Canada: Human Kinetics, 475 Devonshire Road Unit 100, Windsor, ON N8Y 2L5
1-800-465-7301 (in Canada only)
e-mail: humank@hkcanada.com

Europe: Human Kinetics, P.O. Box IW14, Leeds LS16 6TR, United Kingdom
+44 (0)113-278 1708
e-mail: humank@hkeurope.com

Australia: Human Kinetics, 57A Price Avenue, Lower Mitcham, South Australia 5062
(08) 82771555
e-mail: humank@hkaustralia.com

New Zealand: Human Kinetics, P.O. Box 105-231, Auckland Central
09-523-3462
e-mail: humank@hknewz.com

contents

introduction

Before anyone undertakes an exercise program or increases the amount of exercise they are doing, it is the duty of exercise specialists and sports health care providers to make sure that it is safe for them to start or modify an exercise program. This procedure is called *pre-exercise screening*. The aim of the *Pre-Exercise Health Screening Guide* is to introduce professionals in the field to the rationale and procedures for pre-exercise screening. The guide describes the general structure of pre-exercise screening protocols and provides a detailed account of the pre-exercise screening system developed by the American College of Sports Medicine (ACSM, 1995).

The *Pre-Exercise Health Screening Guide* has three chapters. Chapter 1 deals with the need for screening from legal, ethical, and health viewpoints; discusses the risks and benefits of exercising; and asks whether the benefits of screening justify the economic cost. Chapter 2 describes several competing pre-exercise screening systems currently used throughout the world, emphasizing their common overall structure. Most screening systems have a four-part structure:

1. Testing for known disease
2. Testing for signs and symptoms of disease
3. Assessing cardiac risk factors
4. Considering age and exercise intentions

Chapter 2 also points out subtle differences that have in the past led to confusion and uncertainty.

Chapter 3 takes you step-by-step through the most popular of these systems, the ACSM 1995 system. It describes in detail how the ACSM 1995 system works and contains detailed flowcharts that clearly illustrate for you how to apply this screening system.

The appendixes contain reference materials and tools you can use to facilitate your pre-exercise screening process. Appendix A contains a comprehensive screening questionnaire for gathering pertinent screening information from clients and a sample pre-exercise screening report for sharing screening results with clients. Appendix B provides realistic practice scenarios that will help you develop your skills in applying the ACSM 1995 screening system. Appendix C consists of a pharmacopoeia that identifies the common actions of a number of over-the-counter and frequently prescribed drugs.

Familiarizing yourself with the information in the *Pre-Exercise Health Screening Guide* will enable you to

1. understand the legal, ethical, and health implications of pre-exercise screening;

2. explain the benefits of regular exercise in terms of reduced risk of cardiovascular disease, but also appreciate that exercise itself poses dangers;

3. describe the four stages of screening common to many screening systems: assessing for known disease, signs and symptoms, risk factors, and age and exercise intentions;

4. describe the incidence of common risk factors, the interrelationship between risk factors, and the logic of the cut-offs used in the ACSM 1995 system; and

5. screen any individual using the ACSM 1995 system, deciding whether they require a medical check-up before exercise and whether a physician must be present during maximal and/or submaximal testing.

chapter 1

introduction to pre-exercise screening

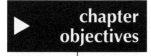

After completing this chapter, you will

1. be familiar with the primary uses for pre-exercise screening systems,

2. understand the appropriate role of sports health care providers and exercise professionals in performing pre-exercise screening,

3. recognize the relative risks and benefits associated with pre-exercise testing and exercise,

4. be aware of the important role a good pre-exercise screening system can play in helping clients avoid unnecessary risks and even death, and

5. understand the importance of pre-exercise screening in selectively identifying people at risk and thus reducing medical costs.

why screen?

Pre-exercise screening can be used

▶ for diagnostic and prognostic purposes,

▶ for exercise prescription,

▶ for performance prediction, and

▶ to motivate individuals.

However, the main purpose of **pre-exercise screening** is to identify and exclude people who may have medical conditions that may put them at risk when they are tested or when they exercise. Despite the fact that injury and death during exercise occur very rarely (Siscovick, 1990; Thompson & Fahrenbâch, 1994), nobody wants to be faced with the situation in which a client suffers medical problems due to inappropriate exercise administration.

Professional associations for exercise specialists, such as the American College of Sports Medicine (ACSM), Sports Medicine Australia (SMA), and the Australian Association for Exercise and Sports Science (AAESS), acknowledge that pre-exercise screening is an important part of the duties of an exercise specialist. This means that if you fail to perform appropriate pre-exercise screening and something happens to a client under your care, a court may find that you have not fulfilled your **duty of care**. Some people think that by having clients sign an informed consent or disclaimer before exercising or testing they can be clear of responsibility. This is not true. You cannot waive or sign away your duty of care.

Pre-exercise screening is part of the duty of care of exercise specialists and ensures that standards of practice are upheld within the profession. Although there is no specific law that says you must conduct pre-exercise screening or how it must be done, you always have a duty of care to your clients. You should also be aware that some forms of personal indemnity insurance—such as that held by many fitness leaders in Australia—only cover "low-risk" individuals.

Unfortunately, awareness of screening issues is very low. A recent study showed that in the United States only 23% of physicians were familiar with the ACSM guidelines regarding exercise prescription. No figures are available for Australia, but anecdotal evidence suggests a very low level of awareness of the guidelines. Recently, there have been cases in Queensland and South Australia of medical doctors refusing to give exercise clearances to people referred to them by exercise professionals (EPs).

A survey that we conducted of screening practices in Australian fitness centers found very little consistency in the way in which pre-exercise screening was administered. Some centers did not use questionnaires at all. Others administered questionnaires but simply filed them without follow-up or further referral. Still others routinely sent all potential members for pre-exercise medical screening. Many of the screening systems used by individual centers have been developed in-house in an ad hoc fashion. Furthermore, there has been no attempt to standardize education and training programs in pre-exercise screening for EPs. This creates a number of difficulties in defining professional practice for the purposes of liability insurance and standardization of referral procedures.

This guide is designed to familiarize EPs and other health professionals with screening guidelines and to clarify the roles and responsibilities of the various players in the exercise and fitness area. You may be thinking that pre-exercise screening should be left to medical doctors. However, there is no law that says that pre-exercise screening has to be performed by a medical doctor. Health professionals are often called on to perform pre-exercise screening as part of their job—in gyms, sporting clubs, exercise testing laboratories, and sports institutes.

In Australia, the Department of the Arts, Sport, the Environment and Territories (DASET) survey conducted on over 2,000 randomly chosen residents of Adelaide found that about 13% of people said they intended to start an exercise program, and a further 31% said they intended to increase the amount of exercise they were currently doing (see table 1.1) (DASET, 1992). Of course, not everyone who says that they will increase the amount they exercise actually does, but even so, each year a lot of people start or intensify their exercise programs. All of these people should be subject to pre-exercise screening.

Table 1.1 Percentage of People Reporting Different Exercise Intentions in Australia	
Don't exercise, and don't intend to start	8.3
Don't exercise, but are thinking of starting	12.9
Exercise a bit, and are thinking of doing more	30.8
Exercise a bit, but are not thinking of doing more	13.1
Exercise regularly, and intend to continue	33.3
Other	1.6
Source: DASET, 1992.	

case study

**Taylor vs. Mobil Oil Corp.
Virginia, USA, 1994**

A health professional working for the Mobil Oil Corporation was conducting a routine examination on an executive of the company. Despite the fact that the executive had experienced signs and symptoms of heart disease (chest pains), the health professional failed to administer appropriate pre-exercise screening. He told the executive that it was safe for him to exercise. A week later, while exercising on his home treadmill, the executive died of a massive heart attack (three major coronary arteries were blocked). The executive's wife filed a wrongful death case against the company and the health professional. In spite of an appeal, the executive's wife was awarded $US 4,000,000.

Source: Herbert, 1996.

The system outlined in this guide is based on a careful reading of the ACSM guidelines. However, because these guidelines are often unclear and there are gaps in the guidelines (for example, there is no complete list of "other diseases") and because of a lack of precision regarding age cut-offs, sedentarism, smoking habits, and premature menopause, there has inevitably been some interpretation involved.

HealthScreen, a pre-exercise screening software program available from Human Kinetics, operationalizes the system described here. It removes much of the subjectivity and many of the problems associated with decision making, and it allows for a more consistent approach among professionals. However, no program can remove the need for informed and intelligent professional judgment on a case-by-case basis.

case study

**Corbett vs. Virginia Mason Hospital
Superior Court Case No. 92-2-28260-7**

In 1992, a physical therapist proceeded with an exercise test despite the fact that during the screening process the client's blood pressure was found to be elevated. Following the test, the patient needed emergency treatment and later required by-pass surgery. The physical therapist was found to be negligent in exercising a duty of care. The judgment was awarded against the therapist.

In the United States in the last 20 years, there have been 19 cases of malpractice litigation associated with exercise testing. Of these, five involved alleged failures in pre-exercise screening.

Source: Herbert, 1995.

risks and benefits

Exercise testing and exercise itself have both risks and benefits. It is the job of the EP to weigh up the risks and benefits and to minimize the danger to those most at risk.

the risks of exercise testing

The risks of cardiac incidents or death during testing depend on the nature of the people being tested and the type of test being conducted. The highest risk situation involves people with known disease who are being given **maximal tests** (i.e., tests where the subject is asked to exercise as hard as they can, until they can no longer continue). The lowest risk occurs when screened subjects are given **submaximal tests** (i.e., tests where the subject only exercises at a level below their maximum).

In Canada, over 1,000,000 people have been given submaximal tests after first being screened using the **Physical Activity Readiness Questionnaire (PAR-Q).** This is a brief seven-item questionnaire asking about signs and symptoms of disease. Among those who proceeded to the test, there have been no deaths. In unscreened populations during maximal tests, on the other hand, the risk may be 50 per million (Shephard, 1988). While questionnaires such as the PAR-Q may be very sensitive (that is, they trap a large proportion of those at risk), they may not be very specific (that is, they also trap healthy individuals).

A number of studies have looked at the incidence of ventricular fibrillation, complications requiring hospitalization, other complications, and death during maximal exercise testing. The results are shown in table 1.2. The values are weighted means from a number of studies conducted in **asymptomatic**, **symptomatic**, and diseased patients. All in all, some 1.3 million tests were conducted in the studies summarized. The results show that the incidence of adverse complications during maximal tests is extremely small, especially in asymptomatic populations.

Table 1.2
Rate of Complications and Sudden Death During Maximal Testing for Various Populations*

	Complications	Hospitalization	Fibrillation	Death
Known CHD			2.0	
Symptomatic	12.0	2.5	1.0	1.0
Asymptomatic		0.2		0.2

Note: Incidents per 10,000 tests.
Source: Bowes, 1998.

the risks of exercise

Exercise brings with it increased risk of injury and sudden death. The risks of cardiac incidents or death during exercise depend on the health status of the people being tested and the type of activity they are involved in. The highest risk occurs among older people who have known coronary heart disease

(CHD) and who are performing vigorous activity. The lowest risk occurs among young, apparently healthy individuals involved in moderate activity.

Table 1.3 summarizes some of the literature on this topic. It is clear that even for the highest risk groups, the risk of sudden death while exercising is relatively small. Even so, we should do our best to identify those most at risk in order to minimize the chance of acute medical problems.

Table 1.3
The Risk of Sudden Death From Various Activities in a Range of Populations

Study	Exercising population	Activity	Deaths (per million participants per annum)
Haskell (1981)	known CHD	rehabilitation center	862
van Camp and Peterson (1986)	known CHD	rehabilitation center	128
Thompson et al. (1982)	active	jogging	66
Vuori (1984)	active	walking	8
		jogging	36
		cross-country skiing	211
		ball games	40
Siscovick et al. (1984)	active	various vigorous activities	56

Note: These figures assume the average person exercises for about 30 minutes three or four times per week.

weighing up risks and benefits

It is clear that when we exercise there is a greater risk of sudden death than when we don't. But the cumulative effects of exercise training also protect us against CHD and sudden death. Can we weigh up the risks and benefits?

Table 1.4 shows the risk of dying during exercise as opposed to while not exercising for both sedentary and active individuals. The risk of dying during exercise is very small. If you exercise for 30 minutes each day four times a week, you could expect to die, on average, after about 48,000 years of exercise (calculated on the basis of the risk of sudden death during typical walking and jogging programs). The protective benefit of exercise far outweighs the risks. You would need to exercise 19.5 hours a day for the risks to balance!

Table 1.4
Risk of Sudden Death During Exercise and While Not Exercising (per 100,000,000 hours)

	Regular exercisers	Nonexercisers
Risk of dying while exercising	21	
Risk of dying while not exercising	5	18

Note: based on data from various sources (cf. Siscovick, 1990).

Studies have quantified the added risk of developing CHD that we incur by not exercising. People who do not exercise have 1.5 to 2.5 times the risk of developing CHD as those who do exercise. This risk is similar to that associated with having a systolic blood pressure (SBP) of 150 mmHg, smoking 20 cigarettes a day, or having cholesterol of greater than 6.93 mmol/L (268 mg/dL) (Powell, Thompson, Caspersen, & Kendrick, 1987).

a cost-benefit analysis

There has never been a rigorous analysis of pre-exercise screening systems that has weighed up the costs of administering the system against the benefits it may have in terms of saving lives.

Exclusion rates for most pre-exercise screening systems (i.e., the percentage of people who need to see a physician before starting or increasing exercise), including the ACSM 1995 system, are surprisingly high across age by gender slices (see table 1.5). Using data adjusted to the general population, 31 to 75% of males and 39 to 67% of females would require medical screening. In some age groups, this rises to between 70 and 100%. Even in the youngest age group, about 25% of all respondents would require screening. This means that one in every four young people should be required to have a medical check-up before being allowed to start exercising. In a group of 260 human movement students screened in 1997-1998, 10 to 15% were excluded using the ACSM 1995 system.

Table 1.5
Percentage of People Excluded (Required to Have a Medical Check-Up and Stress Electrocardiogram [ECG]) at Various Stages of the ACSM 1995 System

	Males	Females
% excluded at		
Stage 1: known disease	20.6	22.6
Stage 2: signs and symptoms	10.1	16.3
Stage 3: risk factors	0–44.4*	0–27.8*
Total	30.7–75.1	38.9–66.7

*Note. The percentage excluded at Stage 3 depends on the assumptions we make about what percentage of people want to undertake vigorous, as opposed to moderate, exercise.
Source: Norton et al., 1996.

At current Medicare remuneration rates, and making conservative assumptions about the effectiveness of screening and the risks of exercise, we have calculated that the cost per life saved—were the ACSM 1995 system to be rigorously applied—would be $US 9,600,000 for males and $US 10,700,000 for females (Norton, Olds, Ly, Gore & Bowes, 1998).

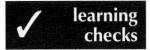

1. Define the following terms:

   asymptomatic

   duty of care

   exclusion rate

   maximal testing

   Physical Activity Readiness Questionnaire (PAR-Q)

   pre-exercise screening

   submaximal testing

   symptomatic

2. How would you explain to a new client who is worried about the dangers of exercise that, while the risk of injury or death transiently increases during exercise, in the long run, exercise is protective against cardiovascular disease? In your answer, you might consider the following points:

   ▶ How much does the risk of sudden death increase while you are exercising?

   ▶ How does the intensity of exercise affect the associated risks?

   ▶ Which populations are most at risk?

   ▶ How does exercise protect against cardiovascular disease in the times between exercise bouts?

3. You are acting as a consultant to a group setting up a chain of fitness centers. Explain to them the benefits of pre-exercise screening systems. In your answer, you should consider

   ▶ the legal liabilities incurred if you don't perform screening,

   ▶ the cost and time involved in performing screening, and

   ▶ other benefits of testing.

the structure of pre-exercise screening systems

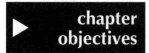

chapter objectives

After completing this chapter, you will

1. be able to compare and contrast different pre-exercise screening systems used throughout the world;

2. understand the stratification of risk categories according to health status;

3. be able to state what constitutes "known disease" in most screening systems;

4. be able to specify signs and symptoms of disease and explain why these signs and symptoms may be markers of disease;

5. be able to list the common cardiac risk factors, including cut-offs commonly used;

6. be familiar with the results of large epidemiological surveys of the incidence of risk factors, the link between risk factors and mortality and morbidity, and the interactions among risk factors;

7. recognize the association between increased risk and age and exercise intensity;

8. be able to set guidelines for moderate and vigorous exercise programs; and

9. recognize the apparent inconsistencies in the choice of cut-off scores for risk factors in terms of death rate.

The purpose of this chapter is to describe the conceptual basis underlying the structure of an effective screening system. This structure is based on the premise that relative risk can be stratified. Those with known disease (Stage 1) are most at risk. Those who do not have known disease but have signs and symptoms that are markers of underlying disease (Stage 2) are at high risk. Those without disease or signs of disease yet who have risk factors suggesting they may develop cardiovascular disease (CVD) (Stage 3) are at increased risk. Apparently healthy individuals who are older and who intend to exercise more vigorously (Stage 4) also are at greater risk.

different screening systems

There are a number of alternative pre-exercise screening systems in use around the world. The ACSM is the largest association for EPs in the world. It has over 15,000 members drawn from more than 72 countries and represents a range of disciplines. The ACSM issued its first edition of pre-exercise screening guidelines in 1975. These were updated in 1980, 1986, 1991, and 1995 and are the most widely used system throughout the world.

In Australia, the umbrella professional association for health professionals is SMA. In 1994, SMA issued pre-exercise screening guidelines based closely on the ACSM 1991 system. At the time, these guidelines were endorsed by AAESS. In 1998, AAESS decided that the ACSM 1995 guidelines should be adopted as the standard for sports health care providers and EPs throughout Australia.

At present in Australia, the ACSM 1991, ACSM 1995, and SMA systems are all occasionally used. All of these systems have been developed by multidisciplinary teams of experts. They are complex and can be quite difficult to interpret, even for experts in the field. While the systems are very similar, the subtle differences can sometimes be confusing.

This guide has followed AAESS in recommending the ACSM 1995 guidelines as the standard. In this chapter and the next, we will provide background information about several key screening issues and outline the ACSM 1995 system.

the four stages of screening

The various pre-exercise screening systems share a common structure, which has evolved since the early 1970s. This structure has four stages, which function like filters or gates that the person who is being screened must pass through. At each stage or gate the person may be excluded—that is, sent to a medical doctor for evaluation—or may pass on to the next stage. Only if the person passes through each stage may he or she be allowed to exercise without a medical check-up and have no medical doctor present during testing.

The four stages of screening include the following:

1. *Known disease*: does this person have any known medical conditions that might endanger them during exercise or exercise testing?

2. *Signs or symptoms of disease*: does this person show signs or symptoms of underlying cardiopulmonary disease, even if it hasn't been diagnosed?

3. *Cardiac risk factors*: does this person have a number of risk factors for heart disease that might mean that they are predisposed to disease?

4. *Age and exercise intentions*: how old is this person, and how vigorously does he or she want to exercise?

stage 1: known disease

The first stage of screening concerns known diseases. **Known disease** includes the following:

▶ *Diabetes.* If the person being screened has had insulin-dependent diabetes mellitus (IDDM) for more than 15 years or is over 30 years old, they are considered to have known disease. If a person has non-insulin-dependent diabetes mellitus (NIDDM) and is over 35, they are considered to have known disease. In Western populations, about 3 to 7% of people are diabetic, of whom about 85 to 90% have NIDDM. Many people have diabetes without knowing it. Exercise may cause very high or very low blood sugar levels in diabetics.

▶ *Cardiovascular disease (CVD).* This includes stroke and heart attacks as well as some other cardiovascular problems, such as blockages in the arteries of the legs.

▶ *Respiratory diseases.* The most common disease in this group is asthma. Asthma is very common, affecting perhaps 5 to 10% of the Australian population. In most cases, asthma is easily controlled by medication, and exercise is not a problem. It is only when people have asthma, are taking medication, and still have breathing troubles that asthma counts as a disease.

▶ *Other diseases.* This category includes liver, kidney, metabolic, mental, or other diseases.

▶ *Pregnancy.* Although not a disease, pregnant women are classified as having known disease for screening purposes.

stage 2: signs and symptoms of disease

The second stage of screening probes for signs and symptoms of disease. Many people have undiagnosed underlying cardiopulmonary disease. Sometimes there are no signs of this at all, but sometimes it is signaled by certain signs or symptoms. Among these **signs and symptoms** are the following:

▶ *Pains in the heart and chest.* This may be a sign of restriction of blood supply to the heart muscle (**ischemia**).

▶ *Shortness of breath,* especially at rest or at night. This may signal reduced blood flow to the lungs, severe lung disease, or heart problems.

▶ *Dizzy spells.* Such spells may be indicative of insufficient blood supply to the brain, or possibly very low blood sugar levels.

▶ *Swelling or accumulation of fluid in and around your ankles (**edema**).* This may indicate an inability of the heart to pump blood around the body.

▶ *Racing or irregular heartbeat (**arrhythmia**).* This indicates electrical problems with the heart.

▶ *Pain in the calves and lower legs (intermittent **claudication**).* This suggests a blockage to the large blood vessels.

▶ *A heart murmur.* This signals either that something is wrong with the valves of the heart or that there is an atrial or ventricular septal defect.

▶ *Undue fatigue.* This may be associated with poor oxygenation of the blood or poor blood flow.

stage 3: cardiac risk factors

The third stage of screening tests for cardiac risk factors. Probing for risk factors serves two purposes:

1. It alerts people to lifestyle risk factors, encouraging them to change their behaviors.
2. It is felt that those who have risk factors of chronic heart disease (CHD) are more likely to have or to develop unrecognized CHD and are thus at greater risk of sudden death during exercise.

The main **risk factors** include the following:

▶ *Age.* In the ACSM 1995 system, this includes men age 46 or older and women age 56 or older at their last birthday. Age is also a risk factor for women under 45 who have experienced menopause and who are not taking hormone replacement medication.

▶ *A family history of CVD.* This means that the person being screened has a parent or sibling who has had CVD before age 55 for male relatives or 65 for female relatives.

▶ *Smoking.* This refers to someone who is currently smoking cigarettes daily or who was smoking regularly within the last two years.

▶ *High blood pressure.* In the ACSM 1995 system, this is defined as having a SBP of greater than or equal to 140 mmHg and/or a diastolic blood pressure (DBP) of greater than or equal to 90 mmHg. Because blood pressure varies a great deal from time to time (particularly because of anxiety at having blood pressure measured!), these pressures must be recorded on at least two separate occasions.

▶ *High cholesterol.* The ACSM 1995 system states that total cholesterol should not exceed 5.2 mmol/L (200 mg/dL).

▶ *Low **high-density lipoprotein (HDL)**.* HDL is the "good" cholesterol. Higher levels of it are better. If HDL is less than 0.9 mmol/L (35 mg/dL) in the ACSM 1995 system, it counts as one risk factor. If HDL is greater than 1.6 mmol/L (60 mg/dL), you actually get a "bonus point"—it can wipe off one other risk factor.

▶ *Diabetes.* As noted previously, in some cases diabetes counts as a known disease, but it can also count as a risk factor (1) if the person being screened has IDDM and either is age 30 or under or has had IDDM for 15 years or less, or (2) if the person has NIDDM and is age 35 or under.

▶ *A **sedentary lifestyle**.* This refers to a person who does no recreational exercise at all *and* has a sedentary job.

Accumulating two or more risk factors may mean that the person being screened should see a medical doctor before starting exercise. Unfortunately, these risk factors are common in the general population, meaning that many people are excluded on the basis of risk factors.

high blood pressure

A 1989 survey in Sydney found that about 82% of men and 88% of women had normal blood pressure. Of the 18% of men who had high blood pressure, it was untreated in about half and treated but uncontrolled in a quarter (see table 2.1). High blood pressure is therefore often undiagnosed.

Table 2.1
Incidence of High Blood Pressure in a Sydney, Australia, Sample (1989)

	Males	Females
Normal blood pressure	82	88
Treated and controlled	5	5
Treated but uncontrolled	4	3
Untreated	9	4

Source: Australian Institute of Health and Welfare, 1996.

Table 2.2
Systolic Blood Pressure (mmHg) Levels From Different Cities and Regions Around the World*

| | MALES | | | | FEMALES | | | |
| | | Percentile | | | | | Percentile | | |
	Number	10th	50th	90th	Number	10th	50th	90th
Catalonia, Spain	397	105	121	146	389	101	118	146
Iceland	657	107	123	146	703	102	118	143
Beijing, China	618	106	126	162	641	102	127	157
Stanford, USA	434	110	127	147	520	105	120	148
Rhein-Neckar, Germany	739	110	128	153	784	104	123	153
Charleroi, Belgium	275	114	129	151	247	107	123	147
Adelaide, Australia	578	111	129	155	565	106	125	149
Sydney, Australia	526	113	130	154	563	107	126	151
North, Sweden	647	112	131	151	614	107	126	154
Auckland, NZ	1,019	111	131	155	568	104	123	150
Belfast, Northern Ireland	927	112	132	163	923	108	129	162
Melbourne, Australia	253	114	133	157	268	105	126	150
Glasgow, Scotland	498	116	134	165	478	109	131	166
Halle, Germany	982	117	137	164	1,055	116	138	172
Pecs, Hungary	605	116	137	166	619	110	134	170
Bremen, Germany	640	118	139	163	658	114	135	168
Turku/Loimaa, Finland	1,199	120	140	168	1,280	114	133	166
Friuli, Italy	713	120	140	170	727	112	136	166
Warsaw, Poland	1,309	119	140	174	1,337	114	138	176
Karelia, Finland	1,144	121	143	169	1,238	118	141	169
Bas-Rhin, France	666	122	143	170	714	113	133	166

*Note: The figures refer to males and females ages 35 to 64 and to data collected between 1978 and 1989.
Source: Australian Institute of Health and Welfare, 1996.

Around the world, blood pressure varies a great deal. It is slightly lower in females than in males. From table 2.2, it is clear that in many countries the median or average SBP is close to the cut-off limit of 140 mmHg used in the ACSM 1995 system. This means that many people will acquire one risk factor through having high blood pressure.

blood lipids

The major blood lipid, or blood fat, we are concerned about is cholesterol. Triglycerides are another form of blood lipid. Elevated triglycerides have been shown to be associated with increased heart disease. Physical activity has resulted in a reduction of triglyceride levels (U.S. Department of Health and Human Services, 1996). Some screening systems take triglyceride levels into account, but the ACSM 1995 system does not. Even though this system does not include a triglyceride cut-off, we recommend that sports health care providers and EPs keep a record of their clients' triglyceride levels, particularly watching for changes over time.

The cut-off levels for cholesterol vary from system to system. Sometimes 6.2 mmol/L (245 mg/dL) is used, sometimes 5.5 mmol/L (217 mg/dL). In the ACSM 1995 system, it is 5.2 mmol/L (200 mg/dL). This is a very strict cut-off and is lower than cut-off levels assigned in ACSM guidelines of previous years. Table 2.3 shows that in only one city in the world, Beijing, is the median cholesterol reading less than the recommended ACSM cut-off. This means that over 50% of adults will acquire one cardiac risk factor based on cholesterol levels. In fact, a survey of Australians conducted by the federal government found that almost

Table 2.3
Total Serum Cholesterol Levels (mmol/L*) From Different Cities and Regions Around the World†

| | MALES | | | | FEMALES | | | |
| | | Percentile | | | | Percentile | | |
	Number	10th	50th	90th	Number	10th	50th	90th
Beijing, China	619	3.3	4.1	5.4	641	3.3	4.2	5.5
Stanford, USA	432	4.2	5.3	6.9	513	4.2	5.2	6.6
Warsaw, Poland	1,289	4.4	5.5	6.8	1,301	4.4	5.5	6.8
Ticino, Switzerland	751	4.3	5.5	6.9	731	4.3	5.2	6.6
Bas-Rhin, France	638	4.3	5.5	7.0	666	4.3	5.4	6.8
Melbourne, Australia	253	4.2	5.6	6.9	268	3.9	5.2	6.9
Darwin, Australia	328	4.3	5.6	6.9	308	4.2	5.0	6.8
Brianza, Italy	616	4.2	5.6	7.1	631	4.2	5.5	7.0
Auckland, NZ	1,005	4.5	5.7	7.0	562	4.5	5.7	7.4
Sydney, Australia	526	4.6	5.7	7.0	563	4.2	5.5	7.0
Rhein-Neckar, Germany	1,158	4.4	5.7	7.2	1,257	4.4	5.7	7.2
Budapest, Hungary	286	4.5	5.7	7.3	565	4.5	5.8	7.4
Belfast, Northern Ireland	916	4.7	5.9	7.4	914	4.7	6.0	7.6
Kaunas, Russia	727	4.7	5.9	7.4	735	4.7	6.0	7.5
Bremen, Germany	627	4.8	6.0	7.7	640	4.8	6.0	7.8
Turku/Loimaa, Finland	1,205	4.9	6.1	7.6	1,280	4.9	6.0	7.8
Ghent, Belgium	415	4.7	6.1	7.7	330	4.7	5.9	7.5
Glasgow, Scotland	464	4.9	6.2	7.7	424	4.9	6.4	8.3
Glostrup, Denmark	1,454	4.9	6.2	7.9	1,359	4.9	6.1	7.8
Kuopio, Finland	977	4.9	6.2	7.9	988	4.9	6.2	8.0
Czechoslovakia	948	5.0	6.3	7.9	990	5.0	6.3	8.0
Karelia, Finland	1,146	5.0	6.3	7.9	1,239	5.0	6.2	8.1

*Note: To convert to mg/dL units, multiply the mmol/L values by 38.7.
†Note: The figures refer to males and females ages 35 to 64 and to data collected between 1978 and 1989.
Source: Australian Institute of Health and Welfare, 1996.

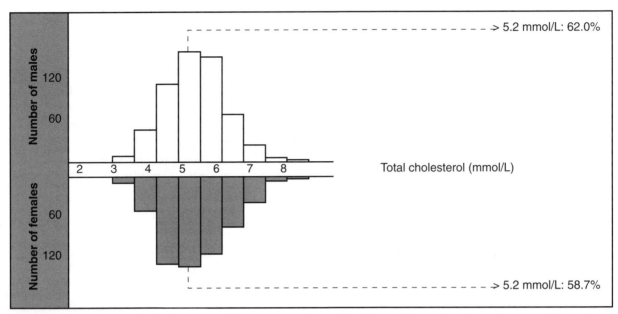

Figure 2.1 Distribution of blood cholesterol levels in Australian adults. About 60% of adults have cholesterol levels above the recommended ACSM 1995 cut-off of 5.2 mmol/L (200 mg/dL).

60% of adults have cholesterol levels above 5.2 mmol/L (200 mg/dL) (DASET, 1992) (see figure 2.1).

Note: Blood lipid measures should be taken after an overnight fast of 8 to 12 hours. Taking food particularly affects blood triglyceride levels but will also elevate blood cholesterol.

Not all cholesterol is "bad." Total cholesterol consists of **low-density lipoprotein (LDL),** which is known to cause heart disease, and high-density lipoprotein (HDL). HDL has been shown to protect against heart disease by scavenging lipid throughout the circulatory system and transporting it back to the liver for processing and elimination. There are some other types of lipoprotein as well, but they are quantitatively unimportant. Figure 2.2 shows data from a large U.S. study (the Framingham study). It shows that the risk of heart disease increases as levels of LDL increase and as levels of HDL decrease.

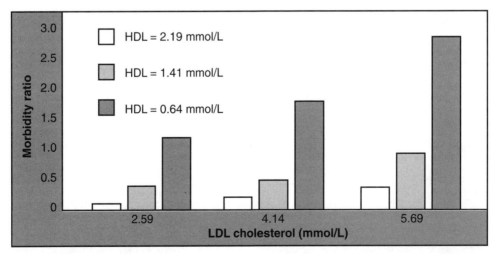

Figure 2.2 The effect of levels of LDL and HDL cholesterol on the risk of heart disease. The vertical axis shows the ratio of the chances of developing CVD relative to the average risk in the population. *Source:* Kannel, 1995.

Usually, when we conduct a blood test we measure total cholesterol. Because the amount of LDL is usually much greater than the amount of HDL, total cholesterol gives us a good idea of how much LDL we have and therefore of heart disease risk. To be able to separate LDL and HDL, we need to use more complex tests. Because HDL protects against heart disease, the ACSM 1995 guidelines award a bonus point—a "positive risk factor"—which can wipe out a negative risk factor if you have HDL levels greater than 1.6 mmol/L (60 mg/dL).

smoking

About 30% of Australians reported smoking cigarettes in the DASET survey (see table 2.4). Smoking is most common in the following groups:

▶ *Younger age groups.* 40 to 50% of people ages 18 to 29 smoke, compared to 10 to 20% of people ages 60 to 69.

▶ *Lower socioeconomic groups.* People from low socioeconomic groups are 1.4 times as likely to smoke as those from high socioeconomic groups.

▶ *Less active people.* Those who do not exercise are 1.27 times more likely to smoke than those who are in the "high activity" category.

Smoking is considered a risk factor not only because of the damage it can do to the lungs, increasing the risk of emphysema and lung cancer. Smoking can also lead to peripheral vascular disease. One of the main causes of amputations is smoking.

Figure 2.3 shows the effect of cigarette smoking on the risk of death from CVD. Cigarette smoking increases the risk for men in every age group. As a rule of thumb, every pack of cigarettes smoked per day increases the risk by 1.5 to 2 times.

Table 2.4
Percentage of Smokers by Gender and Age Group in Australia

Age	Male	Female
18-29	41.2	47.5
30-39	33.0	29.9
40-49	28.2	24.0
50-59	24.4	18.3
60-69	21.4	10.1
≥ 70	18.3	14.4
All ages	29.2	25.5

Source: DASET, 1992.

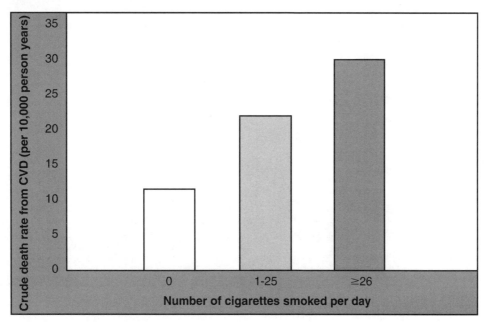

Figure 2.3 Relationship between the number of cigarettes smoked and death rate from CVD for 35- to 57-year-old males.
Source: Neaton and Wentworth, 1992.

sedentarism

Nutritional surveys consistently find that since the beginning of the century, people in both Australia and the United States have been eating less—and eating less fat—and yet obesity has been increasing (U.S. Department of Agriculture, 1994). The obvious conclusion is that people are becoming more sedentary. This is certainly true as regards occupation. There are very few jobs now that demand even a moderate level of physical exertion.

There is also strong evidence that only a small percentage of people undertake recreational exercise at a level sufficient to result in increases in fitness (see table 2.5 and figure 2.4). About 10% of men and 5% of women undertake vigorous exercise (enough to make them huff and puff, or at greater than 60% $\dot{V}O_2$max or about 70% of maximal heart rate) three or more times per week— a level often suggested as necessary for increases in health-related fitness. A further 25 to 30% undertake vigorous exercise, but less than three times per week.

Table 2.5
Activity Levels for Australian Males and Females Ages 18 and Over

	Males	Females
Sedentary	22.4	23.8
Low	30.2	36.6
Moderate	31.8	26.0
High	15.6	13.6

Source: DASET, 1992.

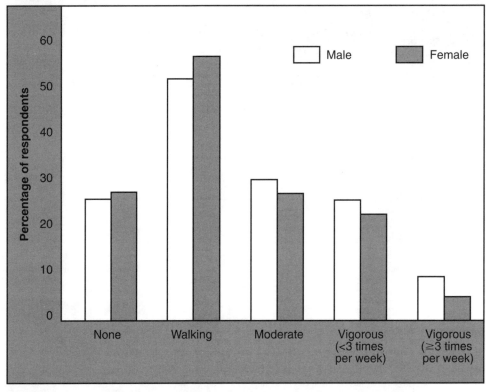

Figure 2.4   The percentage of people undertaking various types of exercise in Australia. These are National Heart Foundation data based on a Melbourne survey, standardized to the World Standard Population.
Source: Australian Institute of Health and Welfare, 1996.

Not surprisingly, levels of activity decrease with age. Whereas 20.4% of males and 21.1% of females ages 18 to 29 are categorized as highly active, only 13.4% of 60- to 69-year-old males and 11.7% of 60- to 69-year-old females fall into that category.

A sedentary lifestyle is recognized as a risk factor for the first time in the ACSM 1995 guidelines. We have defined it as having a sedentary job and doing no formal or structured exercise.

Recent studies have supported the idea that activity levels (or fitness, which is closely associated with activity levels) is an independent risk factor for CVD. From 1970 to 1989, a very large study involving 25,341 men and 7,080 women was conducted at the Cooper Institute. After initial testing, the participants were followed up for an average of eight to nine years. During that period, there were 690 deaths. Deaths and illnesses were noted and related to characteristics such as fitness, blood pressure, and cholesterol levels. Low fitness (being in the least fit 20%) was the third strongest risk factor for death from CVD behind abnormal ECG, chronic illness (males), and high blood glucose (females). Low fitness was a stronger risk factor than high blood pressure, high cholesterol, and a family history of heart disease.

When the characteristics of those who died were compared with those who survived, there were clear differences in fitness levels (see figure 2.5).

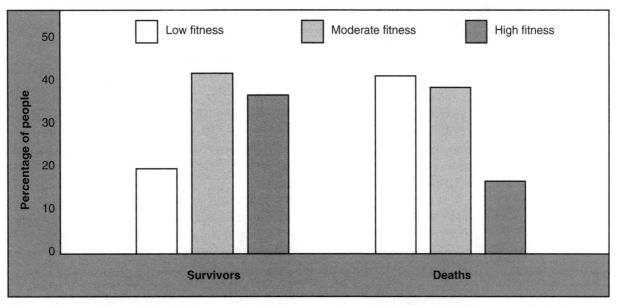

Figure 2.5   Percentages of people with low initial fitness (lowest 20%), moderate fitness (middle 40%), and high fitness (top 40%) among those who died and those who survived during a 20-year follow-up of participants at the Cooper Institute.
Source: Blair et al., 1996.

the relationship among risk factors

So far, we have considered risk factors independently of each other. In reality, there are correlations among risk factors so that if you have one risk factor (e.g., smoking), the likelihood of having another (e.g., sedentarism) is increased. Having multiple risk factors increases the risk of developing CVD

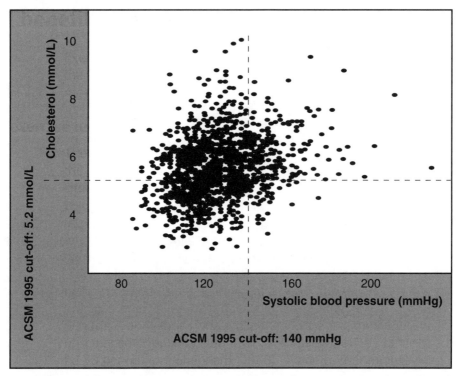

Figure 2.6   Distribution of SBP and cholesterol values in the Australian population, based on data from the DASET survey (1992). The ACSM 1995 cut-off values (140 mmHg and 5.2 mmol/L [200 mg/dL]) are shown.
Source: DASET, 1992.

in complex ways. Figure 2.6 shows the relationship between SBP and cholesterol in Australians. You can see that the datapoints form a cluster that slopes upward to the right. The ACSM 1995 cut-offs of 140 mmHg and 5.2 mmol/L (200 mg/dL) are shown. Anyone in the top right-hand corner already has two risk factors.

Which risk factors are the most important? This depends on how you set cut-off levels for risk factors and the kind of statistical analysis you do. A recent study (Blair et al., 1996) has tried to rank the importance of the risk factors. Risk factors are often expressed in terms of **relative risk**, which is the risk the subject incurs relative to some population standard—for example, the risk a person has of developing CVD if their DBP is greater than 90 mmHg relative to those with DBP of less than 90 mmHg. The results of the Blair study are shown in figure 2.7. If we consider the impact of different risk factors on death from all causes (not just heart disease), smoking, low fitness, and ECG abnormalities are all important, while a high body mass index (BMI) and family history are less important.

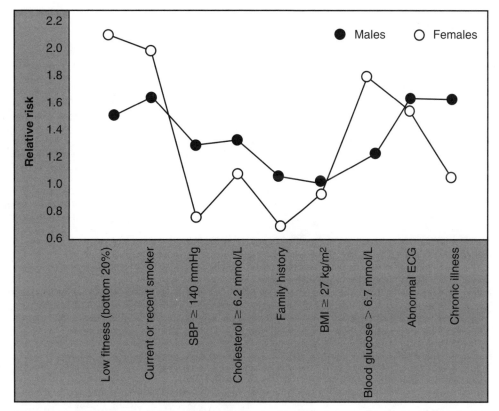

Figure 2.7   Relative risk of all-cause mortality for various risk factors, adjusted for age and other factors, for males and females.
Source: Blair et al., 1996.

◎ case study

Laurent is a 47-year-old taxi driver, who smokes a pack of Gauloises each day and drinks 4 to 5 glasses of red wine. He does very little leisure-time exercise and gets little physical activity on the job. His serum cholesterol concentration was measured earlier this year at 5.8 mmol/L (229 mg/dL), about average for his age. His blood pressure is a little high: 138/92.

Using the ACSM 1995 system, Laurent has at least five risk factors: age, sedentarism, smoking, high DBP, and high cholesterol. Even in the absence of known disease or signs of disease, he is definitely in the "at risk" category.

stage 4: age and exercise intentions

The fourth stage of the screening procedure takes into account the age of the person being screened and their exercise intentions—that is, whether they intend to exercise vigorously (higher risk) or at a moderate intensity (lower risk). **Vigorous exercise** is defined as exercise requiring greater than 60% of $\dot{V}O_2$max (for most people, this means exercise at approximately 70% maximal heart rate [HR]). Using the estimated $\dot{V}O_2$max values from the DASET survey, most 45-year-old subjects could not even jog at 8 km/h (about 5 mph) at 60% $\dot{V}O_2$max. Therefore, for many people, any type of jogging would be vigorous. Table 2.6 identifies the types of exercise activities preferred by Australians according to both gender and age.

Risk of CVD increases with age in both men and women (see figure 2.8). As a rule of thumb, the death rate from CVD doubles with every five-year increase in age from 25 onward. This adds up, so that 65- to 69-year old men are about 436 times more likely to die of CVD than 25- to 30-year-old men. For women, the risk multiplies about 765 times.

Table 2.6
Preferred Activities of Australians by Gender (Top Panel) and Age (Bottom Panel)

Rank	Males	Females
1	walking (41.7)*	walking (57.9)
2	swimming (36.6)	swimming (37.4)
3	cycling (30.6)	aerobics (28.0)
4	weight lifting (26.0)	cycling (22.7)
5	racquet sports (20.4)	weight lifting (14.2)
6	team sports (16.4)	racquet sports (11.2)
7	jogging (15.1)	team sports (9.5)
8	aerobics (5.9)	jogging (6.3)

Rank	< 40 years	≥ 40 years
1	team sports (37.2)	walking (18.3)
2	weight lifting (35.8)	swimming (11.7)
3	jogging (33.9)	cycling (10.2)
4	aerobics (27.7)	aerobics (8.7)
5	racquet sports (27.0)	racquet sports (7.9)
6	cycling (24.2)	jogging (4.7)
7	swimming (22.2)	weight lifting (4.2)
8	walking (11.5)	team sports (4.2)

*Note: The figures in parentheses are percentages of Australians who report that they do these activities to keep fit.
Source: DASET, 1992.

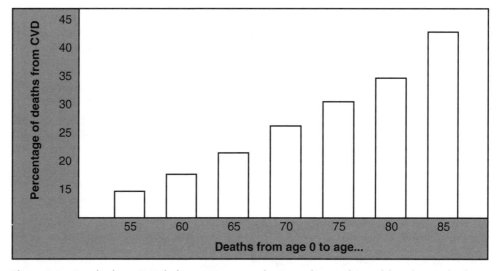

Figure 2.8 Deaths from CVD below various ages for Australian males and females. Only about 15% of deaths below age 55 are due to CVD. Of all people who die before age 85, over 40% of all deaths are from CVD.
Source: National Heart Foundation, 1995.

Age cut-offs have varied over time. The ACSM 1995 system treats men age 41 or over at their last birthday and women age 51 or older at their last birthday differently from younger people. The precise recommendations depend on whether or not they have cardiac risk factors and what type of exercise they want to do. All screening systems have different age cut-offs for men compared to women. This is because risk is much greater for men than for women at all ages (see figure 2.9).

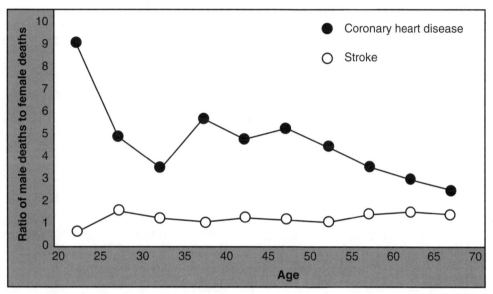

Figure 2.9 The ratio of male to female death rates from coronary heart disease and stroke at different ages (Australian data from 1990-1994).
Source: National Heart Foundation, 1995.

The ACSM 1995 system treats people differently according to whether they want to exercise vigorously or moderately. As stated earlier, vigorous exercise is defined as exercise that elicits greater than 60% $\dot{V}O_2$max. The rationale behind this is that vigorous exercise places a greater strain on the heart, demanding a greater blood flow and oxygen supply to the heart and producing higher blood pressure.

People with cardiac risk factors or who are older (age 41 or older for males and age 51 or older for females) may not require a medical check-up before exercise if they only want to undertake **moderate exercise** (i.e., exercise that elicits less than or equal to 60% $\dot{V}O_2$max). However, if they want to undertake vigorous exercise, they must first see a medical doctor for a clearance.

What does vigorous or moderate exercise mean in practice? This of course depends on the fitness levels of the person being screened. Table 2.7 shows the kinds of work rates that would be equivalent to 60% $\dot{V}O_2$max in average men and women. Any work rate above those given would be classified as vigorous for the average person.

Table 2.7
What Does Moderate Exercise Mean?*

An average 78-kg man of age	20	30	40	50	60	70	
Will have a $\dot{V}O_2$max of	46.4	43.1	39.8	36.6	33.3	30.0	ml/kg/min
60% of $\dot{V}O_2$max will be	27.9	25.9	23.9	21.9	20.0	18.0	ml/kg/min
Will be able to walk at	—	—	—	6.9	6.5	6.1	km/h[†]
Run at	8.1	7.4	—	—	—	—	km/h[†]
Row a Concept II rower at	2:28	2:32	2:37	2:43	2:50	2:57	min/500 m
Ride a stationary bike at	151	138	125	112	100	87	W
Climb on a VersaClimber at	23.2	21.1	19.0	16.9	14.8	12.7	m/min
Corresponding to a HR of	148	142	136	130	124	118	beats/min
An average 65-kg woman of age	20	30	40	50	60	70	
Will have a $\dot{V}O_2$max of	38.3	35.4	32.5	29.6	26.6	23.7	ml/kg/min
60% of $\dot{V}O_2$max will be	23.0	21.2	19.5	17.7	16.0	14.2	ml/kg/min
Will be able to walk at	—	6.8	6.4	6.1	5.6	5.2	km/h[†]
Run at	—	—	—	—	—	—	km/h[†]
Row a Concept II rower at	2:52	2:58	3:05	3:12	3:24	3:31	min/500 m
Ride a stationary bike at	95	85	76	66	57	47	W
Climb on a VersaClimber at	18.0	16.2	14.3	12.4	10.5	8.7	m/min
Corresponding to a HR of	148	142	136	130	124	118	beats/min

*Note: Values that are missing indicate running speeds less than 7 km/h or walking speeds greater than 7 km/h. Concept II figures refer to large cog, vent closed. Exercise of any greater intensity would be classified as vigorous.

[†]Note: To convert from km/h to mph, multiply the km/h values by 0.62137.

how are cut-offs chosen?

Why do we consider a cholesterol concentration of 5.2 mmol/L (200 mg/dL) elevated but 4.8 mmol/L (186 mg/dL), for instance, to be satisfactory? There is no clear answer to this question. In many cases, cut-offs appear to be inconsistent and rather arbitrary. Figure 2.10 shows the relationship between various risk factors and death rate. The cut-offs used by the ACSM 1995 system correspond to death rates ranging from 12 to 25 per 10,000 person years.

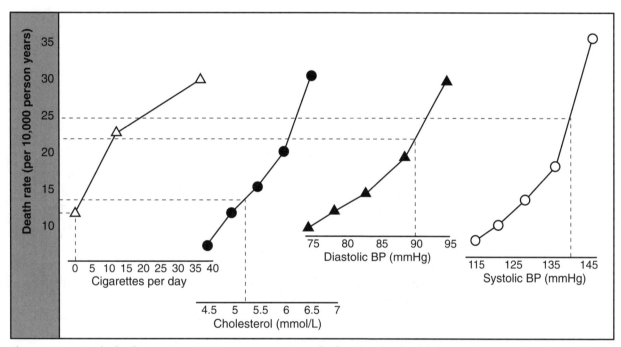

Figure 2.10   Crude death rates (per 10,000 person years) graphed against levels of different risk factors (smoking, SBP and DBP, and cholesterol). The dotted lines indicate the ACSM 1995 cut-offs. You can see that the cut-offs for different risk factors do not always correspond to the same death rate.

Source: Neaton & Wentworth, 1992.

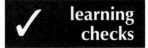

1. Define the following terms:

    arrhythmia

    claudication

    edema

    high-density lipoprotein (HDL)

    ischemia

    known disease

    low-density lipoprotein (LDL)

    moderate exercise

    relative risk

    risk factors

    sedentary lifestyle

    signs and symptoms of disease

    vigorous exercise

2. You are counseling a client about the impact of lifestyle and risk factors on the incidence of heart disease. Which risk factors are the most important from a relative risk point of view? As you think about your response, refer to figure 2.7 on page 21.

3. You are setting up an exercise program for a 50-year-old male. You only want him to exercise moderately (i.e., at no more than 60% $\dot{V}O_2max$). He wants to row using a Concept II rower. What speed should he keep at or below? What heart rate should he try to maintain? Refer to table 2.7 on page 24.

chapter 3

the ACSM
1995 system

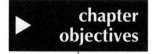

After completing this chapter, you will be able to

1. state the three questions that pre-exercise screening procedures are designed to answer;

2. screen any individual using the ACSM 1995 screening system;

3. decide what to do in the case of missing data, using means or making "high-risk" or "low-risk" assumptions; and

4. counsel clients concerning what steps to follow after pre-exercise screening has been administered.

The ACSM 1995 pre-exercise screening system contains important modifications to the previous ACSM systems. For the first time, age and sedentarism are recognized as risk factors, and a "positive risk factor"—high HDL cholesterol—is introduced. There were also changes to age, blood pressure, and cholesterol cut-offs.

Like other screening systems, the ACSM 1995 system is designed to provide the answer to three questions for every person screened:

1. Does this person need to have a medical check-up and exercise ECG before undertaking exercise testing or an exercise program?

2. Does a medical doctor need to be present during a maximal exercise test?

3. Does a medical doctor need to be present during a submaximal exercise test?

A decision as to whether a person needs a medical check-up must be made before that person undertakes any testing, submaximal or maximal. If a person does need a medical check-up, no testing should be conducted or exercise program prescribed without a written clearance from a medical doctor.

This chapter contains a series of flowcharts that will guide you through the ACSM 1995 system (see pages 29-33). The first chart shows an overview of the system, while the others look at each stage in more depth. In deciding the answers to the three preceding questions, you should work systematically through each stage. Appendix A contains a questionnaire, which is designed to elicit all the information you need in order to make decisions using the ACSM 1995 system.

First, ask whether the person has known disease: diabetes, CVD, severe asthma, pregnancy, or other diseases (other diseases might include metabolic disorders, mental illness, arthritis, etc.—this is often a matter for professional judgment). If they do, then they are excluded. They need a check-up, and a medical doctor must be present during both maximal and submaximal testing.

If the person does have known disease, then screening need not proceed to Stages 2, 3, and 4. If the person does *not* have known disease, then we continue on to Stage 2, deciding whether they have signs and symptoms of disease. These are listed on page 12 (see also the Stage 2 flowchart on page 31). Bear in mind that most of these questions are probing for signs of cardiopulmonary disease. For example, we all experience leg pains at some stage—twinges, cramps, strains, or sprains. But if those pains are characteristic of intermittent claudication—blockage of the blood vessels leading to the lower limbs—then they constitute a sign or symptom of CVD.

If the person answers "Yes" to just one question regarding signs or symptoms, then the judgment is clear: as in Stage 1 exclusions, these people need a check-up, and a medical doctor must be present during both maximal and submaximal testing. We need not proceed to Stage 3.

If they show no signs or symptoms, then we move on to Stage 3: assessing cardiac risk factors. After completing Stage 3, every person must then continue on to Stage 4, regardless of how many risk factors they have. The way they are treated depends on their age, exercise intentions, and risk factor status.

◎ case study

Alberto is now 45 years old, but in his younger days he was a champion distance runner. In fact, he was on the American team for the 10,000-meter race at the Montreal Olympics. He has continued to exercise regularly, running the 10-mile round trip to and from work almost every weekday. Alberto looks after himself: he doesn't smoke or drink alcohol, and his blood pressure and cholesterol levels are low. He has never had any heart problems and feels just fine. In fact, it would be difficult to find a healthier 45-year-old man than Alberto. Nevertheless, according to the ACSM guidelines, Alberto should see a physician if he wants to increase his exercise. This is because he is over the age limit set in Stage 4. Any male 41 or older who wants to do vigorous exercise needs a medical check-up.

See page 40 for a sample letter to the doctor you could use in referring Alberto for a check-up.

system overview

Screening for Risks

Screening Recommendations

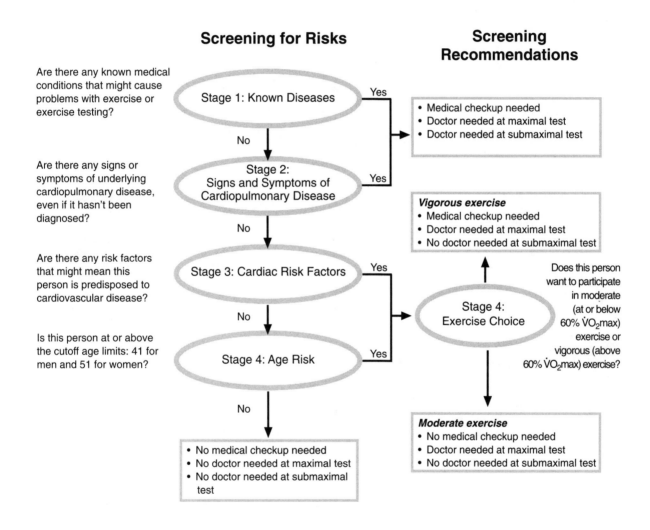

Are there any known medical conditions that might cause problems with exercise or exercise testing?

Stage 1: Known Diseases — Yes

No

Are there any signs or symptoms of underlying cardiopulmonary disease, even if it hasn't been diagnosed?

Stage 2: Signs and Symptoms of Cardiopulmonary Disease — Yes

No

Are there any risk factors that might mean this person is predisposed to cardiovascular disease?

Stage 3: Cardiac Risk Factors — Yes

No

Is this person at or above the cutoff age limits: 41 for men and 51 for women?

Stage 4: Age Risk — Yes

No

- Medical checkup needed
- Doctor needed at maximal test
- Doctor needed at submaximal test

Vigorous exercise
- Medical checkup needed
- Doctor needed at maximal test
- No doctor needed at submaximal test

Stage 4: Exercise Choice

Does this person want to participate in moderate (at or below 60% $\dot{V}O_2$max) exercise or vigorous (above 60% $\dot{V}O_2$max) exercise?

Moderate exercise
- No medical checkup needed
- Doctor needed at maximal test
- No doctor needed at submaximal test

- No medical checkup needed
- No doctor needed at maximal test
- No doctor needed at submaximal test

stage 1: known disease

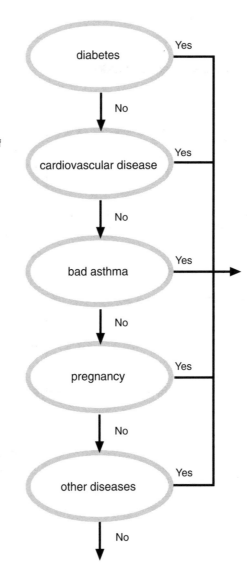

Diabetes counts as a disease if
- this person has IDDM **and** either is > 30 **or** has had IDDM for >15 years **or**
- the subject has NIDDM and is > 35.

A person has cardiovascular disease if
- he has had a stroke **or**
- a doctor has told him he has heart disease **or**
- he is taking cardiovascular medication.

A person has bad asthma if
- she is taking asthma medication **and**
- she answers "Yes" when asked if she suffers from dyspnea or shortness of breath.

A person is classified as pregnant if
- she knows she is pregnant **or**
- she has reason to believe she may be pregnant.

A person is considered to have other diseases if he suffers from liver or kidney disease or other diseases that might prevent him from undertaking physical activity.

diabetes — Yes / No

cardiovascular disease — Yes / No

bad asthma — Yes / No

pregnancy — Yes / No

other diseases — Yes / No

- This person **does** need a medical checkup and exercise ECG before testing or exercise.

- A **medical doctor** must be present during a maximal test.

- A **medical doctor** must be present during a submaximal test.

Proceed to Stage 2: Signs and Symptoms

stage 2: signs and symptoms of disease

Does the subject often have pains in her heart and chest, especially during exercise?

Has the subject at any time in the last 12 months had an attack of shortness of breath that came on during the day when he was not doing anything strenuous?

Does the subject often feel faint or have spells of severe dizziness?

Has the subject had an attack of shortness of breath after exercising at any time in the last 12 months? **or** has he at any time in the last 12 months been awakened at night by an attack of shortness of breath?

Does the subject experience swelling or accumulation of fluid in her ankles?

Does the subject often get the feeling that his heart is beating faster, racing, or skipping beats?

Does the subject regularly get pains in her calves and lower legs during exercise which are not due to soreness or stiffness?

Has the subject's doctor ever told him that he has a heart murmur?

Does the subject experience undue fatigue with usual activities?

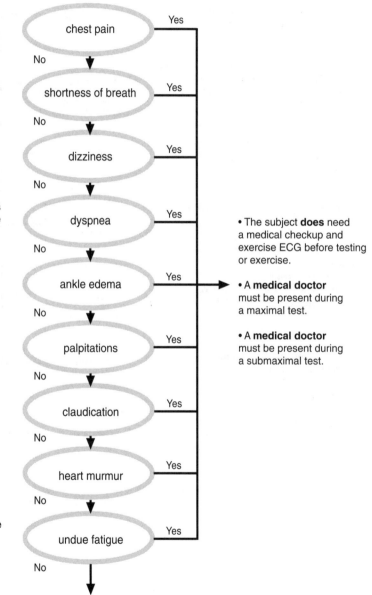

- The subject **does** need a medical checkup and exercise ECG before testing or exercise.

- A **medical doctor** must be present during a maximal test.

- A **medical doctor** must be present during a submaximal test.

Proceed to Stage 3: Cardiac Risk Factors

stage 3: cardiac risk factors

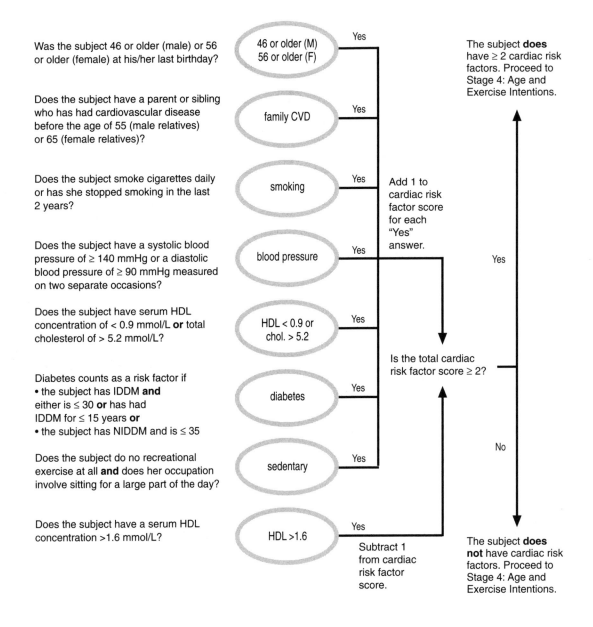

Was the subject 46 or older (male) or 56 or older (female) at his/her last birthday?

→ 46 or older (M) 56 or older (F) — Yes

Does the subject have a parent or sibling who has had cardiovascular disease before the age of 55 (male relatives) or 65 (female relatives)?

→ family CVD — Yes

Does the subject smoke cigarettes daily or has she stopped smoking in the last 2 years?

→ smoking — Yes

Add 1 to cardiac risk factor score for each "Yes" answer.

Does the subject have a systolic blood pressure of ≥ 140 mmHg or a diastolic blood pressure of ≥ 90 mmHg measured on two separate occasions?

→ blood pressure — Yes

Does the subject have serum HDL concentration of < 0.9 mmol/L **or** total cholesterol of > 5.2 mmol/L?

→ HDL < 0.9 or chol. > 5.2 — Yes

Diabetes counts as a risk factor if
• the subject has IDDM **and** either is ≤ 30 **or** has had IDDM for ≤ 15 years **or**
• the subject has NIDDM and is ≤ 35

→ diabetes — Yes

Does the subject do no recreational exercise at all **and** does her occupation involve sitting for a large part of the day?

→ sedentary — Yes

Does the subject have a serum HDL concentration >1.6 mmol/L?

→ HDL >1.6 — Yes

Subtract 1 from cardiac risk factor score.

Is the total cardiac risk factor score ≥ 2?

Yes → The subject **does** have ≥ 2 cardiac risk factors. Proceed to Stage 4: Age and Exercise Intentions.

No → The subject **does not** have cardiac risk factors. Proceed to Stage 4: Age and Exercise Intentions.

32

stage 4: age and exercise intentions

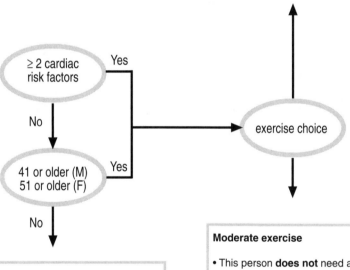

Vigorous exercise

• This person **does** need a medical check up and exercise ECG before testing or exercise.

• A **medical doctor** must be present during a maximal test.

• An **exercise professional** (EP) may conduct a submaximal test.

≥ 2 cardiac risk factors

Yes

No

41 or older (M)
51 or older (F)

Yes

No

exercise choice

• This person **does not** need a medical checkup and exercise ECG before testing or exercise.

• An **EP** may conduct a maximal test.

• An **EP** may conduct a submaximal test.

Moderate exercise

• This person **does not** need a medical checkup and exercise ECG before testing or exercise.

• A **medical doctor** must be present during a maximal test.

• An **EP** may conduct a submaximal test.

how to treat missing information

What should we do if there are missing values—for example, if we can't measure serum HDL? The ACSM system doesn't make any specific recommendations in this case. There seem to be three options:

1. Assume the person is at **low risk**—i.e., assume that missing values do *not* constitute risk factors.

2. Assume the person is at **high risk**—i.e., assume that missing values *do* constitute risk factors.

3. Use **age- and gender-specific population mean values**—i.e., use the average from the best available information.

HealthScreen, a pre-exercise screening software program available from Human Kinetics, allows you to use a scale, or slider, to select from a range of values from low to high risk. If you are not using the software program, you can consult tables 3.1 through 3.4 on pages 35-38. They show age- and gender-specific means, standard deviations, and percentile values for SBP and DBP, total serum cholesterol, and HDL cholesterol for Australian and U.S. populations. You can use these tables to substitute values where values are missing. High percentiles (e.g., 90th percentile) indicate unfavorable values—you would use these if you assume the person being screened is at high risk. Low percentiles (e.g., 10th percentile) indicate favorable values. Use these if you want to assume the person being screened is at low risk. The blood lipid values shown in these tables are for fasting individuals who do not use oral contraceptives.

Table 3.1
Systolic and Diastolic Blood Pressure Means, Standard Deviations, and Percentiles for the Australian Population

SYSTOLIC BLOOD PRESSURE (mmHg)

| Gender | Age | Mean | SD | Percentile | | | | |
				10th	25th	50th	75th	90th
Male	18-24	121	13.1	106	113	121	128	143
	25-34	120	10.3	107	113	120	127	133
	35-44	122	12.0	108	113	121	130	137
	45-54	126	13.9	109	116	126	133	145
	55-64	134	19.0	116	123	131	141	154
	65-74	137	16.5	116	123	137	148	158
Female	18-24	109	11.3	97	101	108	116	122
	25-34	108	11.8	94	101	107	115	121
	35-44	114	12.4	100	106	113	121	131
	45-54	120	13.6	102	110	119	129	138
	55-64	132	17.2	112	118	131	143	152
	65-74	134	12.0	120	126	133	143	148

DIASTOLIC BLOOD PRESSURE (mmHg)

| Gender | Age | Mean | SD | Percentile | | | | |
				10th	25th	50th	75th	90th
Male	18-24	72	9.3	60	67	73	78	83
	25-34	76	8.4	64	70	76	83	86
	35-44	78	9.8	66	72	78	84	90
	45-54	82	9.6	72	77	83	90	96
	55-64	83	10.4	73	77	82	89	95
	65-74	80	9.1	69	73	81	88	93
Female	18-24	67	8.9	56	61	67	74	80
	25-34	67	9.4	55	61	67	74	81
	35-44	73	8.9	62	67	73	80	83
	45-54	76	9.2	65	69	76	83	91
	55-64	81	9.0	69	75	80	88	91
	65-74	80	10.7	70	73	79	84	93

Source: Australian Institute of Health and Welfare, 1996.

Table 3.2
Systolic and Diastolic Blood Pressure Means, Standard Deviations, and Percentiles for the U. S. Population

SYSTOLIC BLOOD PRESSURE (mmHg)

Gender	Age	Mean	SD	Percentile				
				10th	25th	50th	75th	90th
Male	18-24	117	9.6	105	111	117	123	129
	25-34	119	9.9	106	112	119	126	132
	35-44	123	13.9	105	114	123	132	141
	45-54	128	15.4	108	118	128	138	148
	55-64	134	18.0	111	122	134	146	157
	65-74	142	20.1	116	129	142	155	168
Female	18-24	107	8.5	96	101	107	113	118
	25-34	110	10.9	96	103	110	117	124
	35-44	116	14.9	97	106	116	126	135
	45-54	126	17.8	103	114	126	138	149
	55-64	134	19.6	109	121	134	147	159
	65-74	144	20.8	117	130	144	158	170

DIASTOLIC BLOOD PRESSURE (mmHg)

Gender	Age	Mean	SD	Percentile				
				10th	25th	50th	75th	90th
Male	18-24	69	10.0	56	62	69	76	82
	25-34	75	9.4	63	69	75	81	87
	35-44	80	10.5	67	73	80	87	94
	45-54	81	9.7	69	75	81	88	94
	55-64	80	10.0	67	73	80	87	93
	65-74	75	10.8	61	68	75	82	89
Female	18-24	65	8.8	54	59	65	71	76
	25-34	69	9.5	57	63	69	75	81
	35-44	75	10.1	62	68	75	82	88
	45-54	77	9.6	65	71	77	83	89
	55-64	76	9.3	64	70	76	82	88
	65-74	72	10.4	59	65	72	79	85

Source: National Center for Health Statistics, 1994.

Table 3.3
Serum and HDL Cholesterol Percentiles for the Australian Population

TOTAL SERUM CHOLESTEROL (mmol/L)

Gender	Age	Mean	SD	Percentile				
				10th	25th	50th	75th	90th
Male	18-24	4.62	0.87	3.40	3.95	4.56	5.16	5.86
	25-34	5.23	1.15	3.96	4.41	4.97	5.95	6.78
	35-44	5.80	1.08	4.54	5.08	5.78	6.50	7.04
	45-54	5.75	1.09	4.48	5.01	5.67	6.40	7.11
	55-64	5.73	0.96	4.76	5.10	5.72	6.28	7.01
	65-74	5.84	0.91	4.91	5.23	5.75	6.32	7.00
Female	18-24	4.48	0.82	3.45	3.91	4.38	5.21	5.68
	25-34	4.87	0.96	3.78	4.13	4.76	5.53	6.24
	35-44	5.16	0.91	4.16	4.61	5.05	5.66	6.45
	45-54	5.77	1.00	4.46	5.05	5.82	6.33	6.94
	55-64	3.28	1.09	5.09	5.37	6.16	7.04	7.48
	65-74	6.40	0.98	5.28	5.61	6.36	7.21	7.54

HDL CHOLESTEROL (mmol/L)

Gender	Age	Percentile				
		10th	25th	50th	75th	90th
Male	18-24	1.60	1.30	1.09	0.95	0.85
	25-34	1.37	1.25	1.10	0.92	0.77
	35-44	1.51	1.33	1.14	1.01	0.86
	45-54	1.51	1.39	1.09	0.94	0.81
	55-64	1.55	1.29	1.14	0.93	0.85
	65-74	1.47	1.28	1.12	0.96	0.89
Female	18-24	1.66	1.54	1.30	1.18	1.05
	25-34	1.79	1.67	1.39	1.16	1.02
	35-44	1.82	1.54	1.35	1.15	1.00
	45-54	1.87	1.61	1.39	1.11	0.96
	55-64	2.03	1.82	1.50	1.22	1.10
	65-74	1.85	1.59	1.30	1.13	0.98

Source: Australian Institute of Health and Welfare, 1996.

Table 3.4
Serum and HDL Cholesterol Percentiles for the U.S. Population

TOTAL SERUM CHOLESTEROL (mmol/L)

Gender	Age	Mean	SD	Percentile				
				10th	25th	50th	75th	90th
Male	18-24	4.46	0.90	3.30	3.86	4.46	5.06	5.62
	25-34	5.01	0.98	3.75	4.36	5.01	5.66	6.27
	35-44	5.34	1.08	3.95	4.62	5.34	6.06	6.73
	45-54	5.54	1.10	4.13	4.81	5.54	6.27	6.95
	55-64	5.60	1.18	4.08	4.81	5.60	6.39	7.12
	65-74	5.42	1.09	4.02	4.69	5.42	6.15	6.82
Female	18-24	4.58	0.98	3.32	3.93	4.58	5.23	5.84
	25-34	4.84	1.01	3.54	4.17	4.84	5.51	6.14
	35-44	5.05	0.97	3.80	4.40	5.05	5.70	6.28
	45-54	5.60	1.09	4.20	4.87	5.60	6.33	6.98
	55-64	6.05	1.19	4.52	5.26	6.05	6.84	7.56
	65-74	5.99	1.17	4.49	5.21	5.99	6.77	7.47

HDL CHOLESTEROL (mmol/L)

Gender	Age			Percentile				
				10th	25th	50th	75th	90th
Male	18-24			1.65	1.42	1.21	1.03	0.89
	25-34			1.73	1.45	1.20	0.99	0.83
	35-44			1.70	1.41	1.16	0.95	0.79
	45-54			1.70	1.40	1.14	0.93	0.77
	55-64			1.62	1.36	1.13	0.94	0.79
	65-74			1.70	1.42	1.16	0.95	0.79
Female	18-24			1.87	1.60	1.36	1.15	0.99
	25-34			1.92	1.63	1.36	1.13	0.96
	35-44			1.89	1.59	1.32	1.10	0.93
	45-54			1.95	1.65	1.37	1.14	0.96
	55-64			2.04	1.69	1.38	1.13	0.94
	65-74			2.02	1.68	1.39	1.14	0.96

Source: National Center for Health Statistics, 1994.

after screening, what next?

At the completion of the pre-exercise screening evaluation, it is important that clients are appropriately counseled about what the next steps should be. The ACSM 1995 screening system categorizes people according to their risk status. People who are excluded at Stage 1 (known disease) are classified as being in the **Known Disease** category. People excluded at Stage 2 (signs and symptoms) are classified as being in the **Increased Risk (Signs and Symptoms)** category. All people who fall into these two categories need a medical check-up before undergoing exercise testing, and a physician must be present during both maximal and submaximal testing. (See page 40 for a sample letter you can use in referring these clients for a check-up.)

Anyone who is not excluded at Stage 1 or Stage 2, and who has two or more cardiac risk factors, is classified in the **Increased Risk (Cardiac Risk Factors)** category. All others are in the **Apparently Healthy** category. The screening recommendations for people in these categories vary depending on age and exercise intentions. For example, medical check-ups are required for people in the Apparently Healthy category if they are older (41 or over for men and 51 or over for women) and want to exercise vigorously, but not if they are younger. (See the Stage 4 flowchart on page 33 for specific screening recommendations.)

No matter what the screening decision, all recommendations should be seen as equal or parallel paths on the way to a physical activity program. It is important to reassure those clients who *do* need to seek medical advice that this is not a "failure" and that it should not deter them from continuing with their plan to upgrade their physical activity. A medical check-up is done for the client's benefit and should be viewed as a kind of insurance policy. Obviously, it's better to have a check-up ahead of time than to incur unnecessary injury during testing or exercise. Input from their physician can also help ensure the design of their exercise program is tailored to individual needs.

An important aspect of pre-exercise screening is that it helps determine who is best qualified to design and monitor an individual's exercise program:

▶ If the person being screened does *not* need to see a medical doctor, then a suitably accredited fitness leader may design and implement an exercise program and conduct submaximal testing. During maximal testing, however, there may need to be a medical doctor present if this is the screening recommendation.

▶ If the person being screened *does* need to see a medical doctor, a written clearance to exercise must be obtained. For these subjects, exercise programs should be designed and monitored by appropriately qualified professionals (e.g., in Australia, AAESS-accredited exercise physiologists or rehabilitation experts; in the United States, ACSM-certified personnel), although the program may be administered by the fitness leader. If a submaximal test is needed, it is also advisable for a practitioner certified by AAESS or the ACSM to supervise. For maximal testing, a doctor must also be present.

A Sample Letter to the Doctor*

Date: _____

Dear Dr._____:

On _____we screened your patient, _____, using the American College of Sports Medicine (ACSM) 1995 pre-exercise screening system. The ACSM is the largest association for exercise professionals in the world. According to ACSM guidelines, _____ requires a medical examination before undertaking an exercise program. We have provided your patient with a full report showing the screening questions. The screening report indicates any medical conditions, signs and symptoms of disease, and cardiac risk factors that may be present.

_____has indicated an interest in participating in these activities in an exercise program:

Resistance (strength) training:	Yes	No
Vigorous aerobic training (e.g., jogging):	Yes	No
Moderate aerobic training (e.g., walking):	Yes	No
Other training: _____		

In your opinion, is it safe for your patient to participate in the above activities in a prescribed exercise program? If not, please provide comments and suggestions of alternative exercise modes that would be appropriate for_____.

Sincerely,

_____

*Note: The HealthScreen program will automatically offer you the option of printing this letter if your client needs screening.

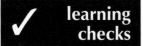

1. Define the following terms:

   age- and gender-specific population mean values

   Apparently Healthy category

   high risk

   Increased Risk (Cardiac Risk Factors) category

   Increased Risk (Signs and Symptoms) category

   Known Disease category

   low risk

2. A client does not know her SBP. She is 37 years old. You decide to use the mean value for her age. Using either table 3.1 or 3.2 (see pages 35-36), decide whether she incurs a risk factor for SBP.

3. George is a 34-year-old male. He has no known disease and no signs and symptoms of disease. He doesn't know what his cholesterol level is, but his blood pressure is okay. He doesn't smoke, but he chews tobacco occasionally. On weekends, George plays ball with his kids, Chester and Max, in the park. George wants to take up an exercise program. He expects to jog at about 10 km/h (6.2 mph) for 30 minutes three times a week. Does George need to see a physician before undertaking an exercise program? As you analyze this case, refer to

   ▶ table 2.7 on page 24, which provides practical information about what counts as moderate exercise;

   ▶ tables 3.1-3.4 on pages 35-38 showing percentile values for blood pressure and blood lipids; and

   ▶ the ACSM screening guidelines.

sample forms

To facilitate the process of pre-exercise screening, we have included a comprehensive screening questionnaire and a pre-exercise health screening report.* The HealthScreen Questionnaire on pages 44-45 is an excellent tool for gathering the information you need to make accurate screening recommendations for your clients. The questionnaire includes questions for each of the four stages of screening: known disease, signs and symptoms of disease, cardiac risk factors, and age and exercise intentions. By obtaining complete and accurate responses to these questions, you can make informed judgments about whether (1) your clients need a medical check-up before undertaking exercise testing or beginning an exercise program, and (2) a physician must supervise maximal and/or submaximal exercise testing.

The Pre-Exercise Health Screening Report on pages 46-47 is a comprehensive report you can use to share information about your screening decisions with clients, their physicians, or other appropriate exercise and health professionals. The report provides clients with a record of their responses to the HealthScreen Questionnaire, a brief explanation of how their responses relate to participating in an exercise program, and the screening recommendation you have made based on these responses. This report is a powerful tool for educating clients regarding the value and relationship of exercise and personal health.

*Note: HealthScreen, the pre-exercise screening software package available from Human Kinetics, contains the HealthScreen Questionnaire and compiles a Pre-Exercise Health Screening Report for each client entered.

HealthScreen Questionnaire

Name _____ Age _____ Gender M F

Address _____

_____ Phone _____

Height _____ Mass _____ Date of test _____

Profession _____

Stage 1—Known Diseases (Medical Conditions)

1. List the medications you take on a regular basis.

2. Do you have diabetes?   No   Yes

   a) If yes, please indicate if it is insulin-dependent diabetes mellitus
   (IDDM) or non–insulin-dependent diabetes mellitus (NIDDM).   IDDM NIDDM

   b) If IDDM, for how many years have you had IDDM?   _____ years

3. Have you had a stroke?   No   Yes

4. Has your doctor ever said you have heart trouble?   No   Yes

5. Do you take asthma medication?   No   Yes

6. Are you or do you have reason to believe you may be pregnant?   No   Yes

7. Is there any other physical reason that prevents you
   from participating in an exercise program (e.g., cancer;
   osteoporosis; severe arthritis; mental illness; thyroid, kidney,
   or liver disease)?   No   Yes

Stage 2—Signs and Symptoms

8. Do you often have pains in your heart, chest, or surrounding
   areas, especially during exercise?   No   Yes

9. Do you often feel faint or have spells of severe dizziness
   during exercise?   No   Yes

10. Do you experience unusual fatigue or shortness of breath
    at rest or with mild exertion?   No   Yes

11. Have you had an attack of shortness of breath that came on
    after you stopped exercising?   No   Yes

12. Have you been awakened at night by an attack of shortness
    of breath?   No   Yes

13. Do you experience swelling or accumulation of fluid in or around
    your ankles?   No   Yes

14. Do you often get the feeling that your heart is beating faster,
    racing, or skipping beats, either at rest or during exercise?   No   Yes

15. Do you regularly get pains in your calves and lower legs during exercise which are not due to soreness or stiffness?   No   Yes

16. Has your doctor ever told you that you have a heart murmur?   No   Yes

Stage 3—Cardiac Risk Factors

17. Do you smoke cigarettes daily, or have you quit smoking within the past two years?   No   Yes

    If yes, how many cigarettes per day do you smoke (or did you smoke in the past two years)?   _____ per day

18. Has your doctor ever told you that you have high blood pressure?   No   Yes

19. Has your father, mother, brother, or sister had a heart attack or suffered from cardiovascular disease before the age of 65?   No   Yes

    If yes,

    a) Was the relative male or female?   _____

    b) At what age did he or she have the stroke or heart attack?   _____

    c) Did this person die suddenly as a result of the stroke or heart attack?   No   Yes

20. Have you experienced menopause before the age of 45?   No   Yes

    If yes, do you take hormone replacement medication?   No   Yes

If known, enter blood pressure and blood lipid values:

21. What is your systolic blood pressure?   _____mmHg

22. What is your diastolic blood pressure?   _____mmHg

23. What is your serum cholesterol level?   _____mmol/L or mg/dL

24. What is your serum HDL level?   _____mmol/L or mg/dL

25. What is your serum triglyceride level?   _____mmol/L or mg/dL

Stage 4—Exercise Intentions

26. Does your job involve sitting for a large part of the day?   No   Yes

27. What are your current activity patterns?

    a) Frequency: _____exercise sessions per week

    b) Intensity: Sedentary   Moderate   Vigorous

    c) History: <3 months   3–12 months   >12 months

    d) Duration: _____minutes per session

28. What types of exercises do you do?

29. Do you want to exercise at a moderate intensity (e.g., brisk walking) or at a vigorous intensity (e.g., jogging)?   Moderate   Vigorous

Pre-Exercise Health Screening Report for

_____

Date of test:_____

This is the report of your pre-exercise screening evaluation. The purpose of this screening is to assist you in safely undertaking an exercise program. The report summarizes your responses to the HealthScreen Questionnaire and provides a recommendation about whether or not it is advisable for you to obtain medical clearance before proceeding with an exercise program. Your exercise professional will help you interpret these recommendations and guide you in the next phase of your physical activity program.

<table>
<tr><td>

Demographic Details

Subject name: _____

Gender:_____

Body mass (kg; lb): _____

Height (cm; in): _____

Age:_____

Profession:_____

</td><td>

Current Exercise Behavior

Exercise frequency: _____

Exercise intensity: _____

Duration of session:_____

History of exercise pattern:_____

Type of exercise: _____

Intended exercise intensity: _____

</td></tr>
</table>

The recent U.S. Surgeon General's report on physical activity recommends that people should try to accumulate at least 30 minutes of physical activity per day on most days of the week. Health benefits can be gained from a variety of activities including brisk walking.

Medical   Your responses

Do you have established, long-term diabetes?   _____

Have you had a stroke?   _____

Do you have heart disease?   _____

Do you have bad asthma?   _____

Do you believe that you are pregnant?   _____

Any other diseases/conditions?   _____

List any medications you are taking.   _____

The preceding questions are included to determine whether there are any known medical conditions that might cause problems when you begin or upgrade an exercise program, or when you undergo an exercise test. If you answer yes to any of these questions it is recommended that, as part of the pre-exercise evaluation, you seek advice from your physician.

Signs and Symptoms   Your responses

Do you experience chest pains?   _____

Have you had episodes of shortness of breath?   _____

Have you had episodes of severe dizziness?   _____

Do you experience dyspnea (breathing difficulty)?   _____

Do you experience ankle edema (swelling in and around your ankles)?   _____

Have you ever had heart palpitations (unusual heart racing/pounding)? _____

Do you regularly get claudication (sharp pains in your legs)?   _____

Has your doctor told you that you have a heart murmur?   _____

Do you experience undue fatigue?   _____

The preceding questions are included to determine whether there are any signs and/or symptoms of underlying cardiopulmonary disease, even if it hasn't been diagnosed. If you answered yes to any of these questions it is recommended that, as part of the pre-exercise evaluation, you seek advice from your physician.

Cardiovascular Risk Factors	Your values	Risk factor limits
Family member with cardiovascular disease?	_____	
Smoking habit?	_____	
Systolic blood pressure (mmHg)*:	_____	140 or greater
Diastolic blood pressure (mmHg)*:	_____	90 or greater
Total cholesterol (mmol/L; mg/dL)*:	_____	greater than 5.2; 200
HDL cholesterol (mmol/L; mg/dL)*:	_____	less than 0.9; 35
Triglycerides (mmol/L; mg/dL)*:	_____	
Diabetes as a risk factor?	_____	
Sedentary lifestyle?	_____	
Premature menopause?	_____	

The preceding questions, together with the measurements taken, have been included to determine whether there are any risk factors that might mean you are predisposed to cardiovascular disease. In the case of HDL cholesterol, the higher the value the better.

The risk factor limits shown indicate the recommended cut-offs where the risk of developing cardiovascular disease significantly increases. Having risk factors may mean that you need to seek medical clearance. This depends on your age and exercise intentions. Advice about how to reduce risk factors is available from your exercise professional or physician.

According to the ACSM guidelines, you are in the following category:

☐ Known disease   ☐ Increased risk (cardiac risk factors)

☐ Increased risk (signs and symptoms)   ☐ Apparently healthy

The overall recommendations for _____ **are as follows:**

(insert client name)

Known Disease or Increased Risk (Signs and Symptoms):

☐ You need a medical check-up and exercise ECG before testing or exercise

   A physician must conduct a maximal exercise test

   A physician must conduct submaximal exercise testing

Increased Risk (Cardiac Risk Factors) or Apparently Healthy—Older (≥ 41 for males, ≥ 51 for females):

Vigorous exercise intended   ☐ You need a medical check-up and exercise ECG before testing or exercise

   A physician must conduct a maximal exercise test

   An exercise professional may conduct submaximal exercise testing

Moderate exercise intended   ☐ You do NOT need a medical check-up and exercise ECG before testing or exercise

   A physician must conduct a maximal exercise test

   An exercise professional may conduct submaximal exercise testing

Apparently Healthy—Younger (< 41 for males, < 51 for females):

☐ You do NOT need a medical check-up and exercise ECG before testing or exercise

   An exercise professional may conduct a maximal exercise test

   An exercise professional may conduct submaximal exercise testing

Signature _____Date_____

Witness _____Date_____

Comments:_____

* Default values based on population norms may have been substituted for missing data.

practice cases

To give you some practice using the ACSM 1995 screening system, we have included several sample questionnaires. Use the information in each of the questionnaires to apply the pre-exercise screening procedure. The questionnaires have been specially designed to supply all the information you will need to make a screening judgment.

Remember that pre-exercise screening asks you to make just three decisions:

1. Does the person being screened need to see a medical doctor and have a stress ECG before undertaking exercise testing or starting an exercise program?

2. Does the person being screened need to have a medical doctor present if they want to have a maximal test, or can an EP conduct the test?

3. Does the person being screened need to have a medical doctor present if they want to have a submaximal text, or can an EP conduct the test?

In many cases, screening decisions are not entirely mechanical. The "other diseases" category, for example, asks you to exercise professional judgment. Some diseases may pose very little exercise risk; others may be unfamiliar and even experts would not be sure of exercise interactions. If in doubt, you should seek the advice of a medical or exercise professional. In most cases, common sense is the best guide.

Evaluate the questionnaire responses by referring to the flowcharts that outline the ACSM 1995 system (see pages 29-33). Move first through each of the items in "Stage 1: Known Disease." If the person being screened does not have known disease, move on to "Stage 2: Signs and Symptoms of Disease," then to "Stage 3: Cardiac Risk Factors," and finally to "Stage 4: Age and Exercise Intentions." Where blood pressure and blood lipid values are missing, refer to tables 3.1-3.4 on pages 35-38 to insert mean values for the person's age and gender. When you have made a screening decision, compare your evaluation with that provided in the "Screening Judgments" section on pages 70-72.

HealthScreen Questionnaire

Name _Annabelle Mant_   **Age** _29_   **Gender**   M   (F)

Address _____

_____ **Phone** _____

Height _64.4 in (163.6 cm)_ **Mass** _126 lb (57.1 kg)_   **Date of test** _____

Profession _taxidermist_ _____

Stage 1—Known Diseases (Medical Conditions)

1. List the medications you take on a regular basis.   _contraceptives_

2. Do you have diabetes?   (No)   Yes

    a) If yes, please indicate if it is insulin-dependent diabetes mellitus (IDDM) or non–insulin-dependent diabetes mellitus (NIDDM).   IDDM   NIDDM

    b) If IDDM, for how many years have you had IDDM?   _____ years

3. Have you had a stroke?   (No)   Yes

4. Has your doctor ever said you have heart trouble?   (No)   Yes

5. Do you take asthma medication?   (No)   Yes

6. Are you or do you have reason to believe you may be pregnant?   (No)   Yes

7. Is there any other physical reason that prevents you from participating in an exercise program (e.g., cancer; osteoporosis; severe arthritis; mental illness; thyroid, kidney, or liver disease)?   (No)   Yes

Stage 2—Signs and Symptoms

8. Do you often have pains in your heart, chest, or surrounding areas, especially during exercise?   (No)   Yes

9. Do you often feel faint or have spells of severe dizziness during exercise?   (No)   Yes

10. Do you experience unusual fatigue or shortness of breath at rest or with mild exertion?   (No)   Yes

11. Have you had an attack of shortness of breath that came on after you stopped exercising?   (No)   Yes

12. Have you been awakened at night by an attack of shortness of breath?   (No)   Yes

13. Do you experience swelling or accumulation of fluid in or around your ankles?   (No)   Yes

14. Do you often get the feeling that your heart is beating faster, racing, or skipping beats, either at rest or during exercise?   (No)   Yes

15. Do you regularly get pains in your calves and lower legs during exercise which are not due to soreness or stiffness? (No) Yes

16. Has your doctor ever told you that you have a heart murmur? (No) Yes

Stage 3—Cardiac Risk Factors

17. Do you smoke cigarettes daily, or have you quit smoking within the past two years? (No) Yes

    If yes, how many cigarettes per day do you smoke (or did you smoke in the past two years)? _____ per day

18. Has your doctor ever told you that you have high blood pressure? (No) Yes

19. Has your father, mother, brother, or sister had a heart attack or suffered from cardiovascular disease before the age of 65? (No) Yes

    If yes,

    a) Was the relative male or female? _____

    b) At what age did he or she have the stroke or heart attack? _____

    c) Did this person die suddenly as a result of the stroke or heart attack? No Yes

20. Have you experienced menopause before the age of 45? (No) Yes

    If yes, do you take hormone replacement medication? No Yes

If known, enter blood pressure and blood lipid values:

21. What is your systolic blood pressure? ____–____ mmHg

22. What is your diastolic blood pressure? __70__ mmHg

23. What is your serum cholesterol level? __4.93__ (mmol/L) or mg/dL

24. What is your serum HDL level? __1.22__ (mmol/L) or mg/dL

25. What is your serum triglyceride level? ____–____ mmol/L or mg/dL

Stage 4—Exercise Intentions

26. Does your job involve sitting for a large part of the day? No (Yes)

27. What are your current activity patterns?

    a) Frequency: __1__ exercise sessions per week

    b) Intensity: Sedentary (Moderate) Vigorous

    c) History: <3 months (3–12 months) >12 months

    d) Duration: __30__ minutes per session

28. What types of exercises do you do? *walking*

29. Do you want to exercise at a moderate intensity (e.g., brisk walking) or at a vigorous intensity (e.g., jogging)? (Moderate) Vigorous

HealthScreen Questionnaire

Name Karma Pope   **Age** 61   **Gender** M (F)

Address _____

_____ **Phone** _____

Height 64.1 in (163 cm)   **Mass** 149 lb (67.6 kg)   **Date of test** _____

Profession biochemist _____

Stage 1—Known Diseases (Medical Conditions)

1. List the medications you take on a regular basis.   **Ventolin Inhaler**

2. Do you have diabetes?   (No)   Yes

   a) If yes, please indicate if it is insulin-dependent diabetes mellitus (IDDM) or non–insulin-dependent diabetes mellitus (NIDDM).   IDDM   NIDDM

   b) If IDDM, for how many years have you had IDDM?   _____ years

3. Have you had a stroke?   (No)   Yes

4. Has your doctor ever said you have heart trouble?   (No)   Yes

5. Do you take asthma medication?   No   (Yes)

6. Are you or do you have reason to believe you may be pregnant?   (No)   Yes

7. Is there any other physical reason that prevents you from participating in an exercise program (e.g., cancer; osteoporosis; severe arthritis; mental illness; thyroid, kidney, or liver disease)?   (No)   Yes

Stage 2—Signs and Symptoms

8. Do you often have pains in your heart, chest, or surrounding areas, especially during exercise?   (No)   Yes

9. Do you often feel faint or have spells of severe dizziness during exercise?   (No)   Yes

10. Do you experience unusual fatigue or shortness of breath at rest or with mild exertion?   No   (Yes)

11. Have you had an attack of shortness of breath that came on after you stopped exercising?   (No)   Yes

12. Have you been awakened at night by an attack of shortness of breath?   (No)   Yes

13. Do you experience swelling or accumulation of fluid in or around your ankles?   (No)   Yes

14. Do you often get the feeling that your heart is beating faster, racing, or skipping beats, either at rest or during exercise?   (No)   Yes

15. Do you regularly get pains in your calves and lower legs during exercise which are not due to soreness or stiffness? (No) Yes

16. Has your doctor ever told you that you have a heart murmur? (No) Yes

Stage 3—Cardiac Risk Factors

17. Do you smoke cigarettes daily, or have you quit smoking within the past two years? (No) Yes

    If yes, how many cigarettes per day do you smoke (or did you smoke in the past two years)? _____ per day

18. Has your doctor ever told you that you have high blood pressure? (No) Yes

19. Has your father, mother, brother, or sister had a heart attack or suffered from cardiovascular disease before the age of 65? (No) Yes

    If yes,

    a) Was the relative male or female? _____

    b) At what age did he or she have the stroke or heart attack? _____

    c) Did this person die suddenly as a result of the stroke or heart attack? No Yes

20. Have you experienced menopause before the age of 45? (No) Yes

    If yes, do you take hormone replacement medication? No Yes

If known, enter blood pressure and blood lipid values:

21. What is your systolic blood pressure? _138_ mmHg

22. What is your diastolic blood pressure? _78_ mmHg

23. What is your serum cholesterol level? _6.22_ (mmol/L) or mg/dL

24. What is your serum HDL level? _—_ mmol/L or mg/dL

25. What is your serum triglyceride level? _—_ mmol/L or mg/dL

Stage 4—Exercise Intentions

26. Does your job involve sitting for a large part of the day? No (Yes)

27. What are your current activity patterns?

    a) Frequency: _1_ exercise sessions per week

    b) Intensity: Sedentary (Moderate) Vigorous

    c) History: <3 months (3–12 months) >12 months

    d) Duration: _30_ minutes per session

28. What types of exercises do you do? **walking**

29. Do you want to exercise at a moderate intensity (e.g., brisk walking) or at a vigorous intensity (e.g., jogging)? Moderate (Vigorous)

HealthScreen Questionnaire

Name Dougall Thompson _____ **Age** 41 _____ **Gender** Ⓜ F

Address _____

_____ **Phone** _____

Height 77.9 in (198 cm) **Mass** 174 lb (79 kg) **Date of test** _____

Profession receptionist _____

Stage 1—Known Diseases (Medical Conditions)

1. List the medications you take on a regular basis. Aspirin

2. Do you have diabetes?   (No)   Yes
   a) If yes, please indicate if it is insulin-dependent diabetes mellitus
      (IDDM) or non–insulin-dependent diabetes mellitus (NIDDM).   IDDM NIDDM
   b) If IDDM, for how many years have you had IDDM?   _____ years

3. Have you had a stroke?   (No)   Yes

4. Has your doctor ever said you have heart trouble?   (No)   Yes

5. Do you take asthma medication?   (No)   Yes

6. Are you or do you have reason to believe you may be pregnant?   (No)   Yes

7. Is there any other physical reason that prevents you
   from participating in an exercise program (e.g., cancer;
   osteoporosis; severe arthritis; mental illness; thyroid, kidney,
   or liver disease)?   (No)   Yes

Stage 2—Signs and Symptoms

8. Do you often have pains in your heart, chest, or surrounding
   areas, especially during exercise?   (No)   Yes

9. Do you often feel faint or have spells of severe dizziness
   during exercise?   (No)   Yes

10. Do you experience unusual fatigue or shortness of breath
    at rest or with mild exertion?   (No)   Yes

11. Have you had an attack of shortness of breath that came on
    after you stopped exercising?   (No)   Yes

12. Have you been awakened at night by an attack of shortness
    of breath?   (No)   Yes

13. Do you experience swelling or accumulation of fluid in or around
    your ankles?   (No)   Yes

14. Do you often get the feeling that your heart is beating faster,
    racing, or skipping beats, either at rest or during exercise?   (No)   Yes

15. Do you regularly get pains in your calves and lower legs during exercise which are not due to soreness or stiffness?   (No)   Yes

16. Has your doctor ever told you that you have a heart murmur?   (No)   Yes

Stage 3—Cardiac Risk Factors

17. Do you smoke cigarettes daily, or have you quit smoking within the past two years?   (No)   Yes

    If yes, how many cigarettes per day do you smoke (or did you smoke in the past two years)?   _____ per day

18. Has your doctor ever told you that you have high blood pressure?   (No)   Yes

19. Has your father, mother, brother, or sister had a heart attack or suffered from cardiovascular disease before the age of 65?   (No)   Yes

    If yes,

    a) Was the relative male or female?   _____

    b) At what age did he or she have the stroke or heart attack?   _____

    c) Did this person die suddenly as a result of the stroke or heart attack?   No   Yes

20. Have you experienced menopause before the age of 45?   No   Yes

    If yes, do you take hormone replacement medication?   No   Yes

If known, enter blood pressure and blood lipid values:

21. What is your systolic blood pressure?   _138_ mmHg

22. What is your diastolic blood pressure?   _84_ mmHg

23. What is your serum cholesterol level?   _5.67_ (mmol/L) or mg/dL

24. What is your serum HDL level?   _1.27_ (mmol/L) or mg/dL

25. What is your serum triglyceride level?   _−_ mmol/L or mg/dL

Stage 4—Exercise Intentions

26. Does your job involve sitting for a large part of the day?   No   (Yes)

27. What are your current activity patterns?

    a) Frequency: _Nil_ exercise sessions per week

    b) Intensity: Sedentary   Moderate   Vigorous

    c) History: <3 months   3–12 months   >12 months

    d) Duration: _____ minutes per session

28. What types of exercises do you do?

29. Do you want to exercise at a moderate intensity (e.g., brisk walking) or at a vigorous intensity (e.g., jogging)?   (Moderate)   Vigorous

HealthScreen Questionnaire

Name _Alanna Ethridge_   **Age** _24_   **Gender**   M Ⓕ

Address _____

_____ **Phone** _____

Height _64.4 in (163.7 cm)_ **Mass** _165 lb (74.9 kg)_ **Date of test** _____

Profession _astronomer_ _____

Stage 1—Known Diseases (Medical Conditions)

1. List the medications you take on a regular basis.   _ventolin inhaler_

2. Do you have diabetes?   (No)   Yes

    a) If yes, please indicate if it is insulin-dependent diabetes mellitus (IDDM) or non–insulin-dependent diabetes mellitus (NIDDM).   IDDM   NIDDM

    b) If IDDM, for how many years have you had IDDM?   _____ years

3. Have you had a stroke?   (No)   Yes

4. Has your doctor ever said you have heart trouble?   (No)   Yes

5. Do you take asthma medication?   (No)   Yes

6. Are you or do you have reason to believe you may be pregnant?   (No)   Yes

7. Is there any other physical reason that prevents you from participating in an exercise program (e.g., cancer; osteoporosis; severe arthritis; mental illness; thyroid, kidney, or liver disease)?   (No)   Yes

Stage 2—Signs and Symptoms

8. Do you often have pains in your heart, chest, or surrounding areas, especially during exercise?   (No)   Yes

9. Do you often feel faint or have spells of severe dizziness during exercise?   (No)   Yes

10. Do you experience unusual fatigue or shortness of breath at rest or with mild exertion?   (No)   Yes

11. Have you had an attack of shortness of breath that came on after you stopped exercising?   (No)   Yes

12. Have you been awakened at night by an attack of shortness of breath?   (No)   Yes

13. Do you experience swelling or accumulation of fluid in or around your ankles?   (No)   Yes

14. Do you often get the feeling that your heart is beating faster, racing, or skipping beats, either at rest or during exercise?   (No)   Yes

15. Do you regularly get pains in your calves and lower legs during exercise which are not due to soreness or stiffness? (No) Yes

16. Has your doctor ever told you that you have a heart murmur? (No) Yes

Stage 3—Cardiac Risk Factors

17. Do you smoke cigarettes daily, or have you quit smoking within the past two years? No (Yes)

    If yes, how many cigarettes per day do you smoke (or did you smoke in the past two years)? _24_ per day

18. Has your doctor ever told you that you have high blood pressure? (No) Yes

19. Has your father, mother, brother, or sister had a heart attack or suffered from cardiovascular disease before the age of 65? No (Yes)

    If yes,

    a) Was the relative male or female? _female_

    b) At what age did he or she have the stroke or heart attack? _44_

    c) Did this person die suddenly as a result of the stroke or heart attack? No (Yes)

20. Have you experienced menopause before the age of 45? (No) Yes

    If yes, do you take hormone replacement medication? No Yes

If known, enter blood pressure and blood lipid values:

21. What is your systolic blood pressure? _104_ mmHg

22. What is your diastolic blood pressure? _84_ mmHg

23. What is your serum cholesterol level? _4.7_ (mmol/L) or mg/dL

24. What is your serum HDL level? _1.43_ (mmol/L) or mg/dL

25. What is your serum triglyceride level? _–_ mmol/L or mg/dL

Stage 4—Exercise Intentions

26. Does your job involve sitting for a large part of the day? No (Yes)

27. What are your current activity patterns?

    a) Frequency: _Nil_ exercise sessions per week

    b) Intensity: Sedentary   Moderate   Vigorous

    c) History: <3 months   3–12 months   >12 months

    d) Duration: _____minutes per session

28. What types of exercises do you do?

29. Do you want to exercise at a moderate intensity (e.g., brisk walking) or at a vigorous intensity (e.g., jogging)? Moderate (Vigorous)

HealthScreen Questionnaire

Name _Vernon Ingleson_ _____   Age __71___   Gender (M) F

Address _____

_____ Phone _____

Height _69.4 in (176.2 cm)_ Mass _137 lb (62.1 kg)__ Date of test _____

Profession _retired_ _____

Stage 1—Known Diseases (Medical Conditions)

1. List the medications you take on a regular basis. **none**

2. Do you have diabetes?   (No)   Yes
    a) If yes, please indicate if it is insulin-dependent diabetes mellitus
       (IDDM) or non–insulin-dependent diabetes mellitus (NIDDM).   IDDM NIDDM
    b) If IDDM, for how many years have you had IDDM?   _____ years

3. Have you had a stroke?   (No)   Yes

4. Has your doctor ever said you have heart trouble?   (No)   Yes

5. Do you take asthma medication?   (No)   Yes

6. Are you or do you have reason to believe you may be pregnant?   (No)   Yes

7. Is there any other physical reason that prevents you
    from participating in an exercise program (e.g., cancer;
    osteoporosis; severe arthritis; mental illness; thyroid, kidney,
    or liver disease)?   (No)   Yes

Stage 2—Signs and Symptoms

8. Do you often have pains in your heart, chest, or surrounding
    areas, especially during exercise?   (No)   Yes

9. Do you often feel faint or have spells of severe dizziness
    during exercise?   (No)   Yes

10. Do you experience unusual fatigue or shortness of breath
    at rest or with mild exertion?   (No)   Yes

11. Have you had an attack of shortness of breath that came on
    after you stopped exercising?   (No)   Yes

12. Have you been awakened at night by an attack of shortness
    of breath?   (No)   Yes

13. Do you experience swelling or accumulation of fluid in or around
    your ankles?   (No)   Yes

14. Do you often get the feeling that your heart is beating faster,
    racing, or skipping beats, either at rest or during exercise?   (No)   Yes

15. Do you regularly get pains in your calves and lower legs during exercise which are not due to soreness or stiffness?   (No)   Yes

16. Has your doctor ever told you that you have a heart murmur?   (No)   Yes

Stage 3—Cardiac Risk Factors

17. Do you smoke cigarettes daily, or have you quit smoking within the past two years?   (No)   Yes

    If yes, how many cigarettes per day do you smoke (or did you smoke in the past two years)?   _____ per day

18. Has your doctor ever told you that you have high blood pressure?   (No)   Yes

19. Has your father, mother, brother, or sister had a heart attack or suffered from cardiovascular disease before the age of 65?   (No)   Yes

    If yes,

    a) Was the relative male or female?   _____

    b) At what age did he or she have the stroke or heart attack?   _____

    c) Did this person die suddenly as a result of the stroke or heart attack?   No   Yes

20. Have you experienced menopause before the age of 45?   No   Yes

    If yes, do you take hormone replacement medication?   No   Yes

If known, enter blood pressure and blood lipid values:

21. What is your systolic blood pressure?   __165__ mmHg

22. What is your diastolic blood pressure?   __78__ mmHg

23. What is your serum cholesterol level?   __6.2__ (mmol/L) or mg/dL

24. What is your serum HDL level?   __0.85__ (mmol/L) or mg/dL

25. What is your serum triglyceride level?   __—__ mmol/L or mg/dL

Stage 4—Exercise Intentions

26. Does your job involve sitting for a large part of the day?   No   (Yes)

27. What are your current activity patterns?

    a) Frequency: __Nil__ exercise sessions per week

    b) Intensity: Sedentary   Moderate   Vigorous

    c) History: <3 months   3–12 months   >12 months

    d) Duration: _____ minutes per session

28. What types of exercises do you do?

29. Do you want to exercise at a moderate intensity (e.g., brisk walking) or at a vigorous intensity (e.g., jogging)?   Moderate   (Vigorous)

HealthScreen Questionnaire

Name *Sabine Andrews*   **Age** *40*   **Gender**   M ⓕ

Address _____

_____ **Phone** _____

Height *64 in (162.6 cm)*   **Mass** *187 lb (84.9 kg)*   **Date of test** _____

Profession *Home duties* _____

Stage 1—Known Diseases (Medical Conditions)

1. List the medications you take on a regular basis.   *Premarin*

2. Do you have diabetes?   (No)   Yes

    a) If yes, please indicate if it is insulin-dependent diabetes mellitus
       (IDDM) or non–insulin-dependent diabetes mellitus (NIDDM).   IDDM   NIDDM

    b) If IDDM, for how many years have you had IDDM?   _____ years

3. Have you had a stroke?   (No)   Yes

4. Has your doctor ever said you have heart trouble?   (No)   Yes

5. Do you take asthma medication?   (No)   Yes

6. Are you or do you have reason to believe you may be pregnant?   (No)   Yes

7. Is there any other physical reason that prevents you
from participating in an exercise program (e.g., cancer;
osteoporosis; severe arthritis; mental illness; thyroid, kidney,
or liver disease)?   (No)   Yes

Stage 2—Signs and Symptoms

8. Do you often have pains in your heart, chest, or surrounding
areas, especially during exercise?   (No)   Yes

9. Do you often feel faint or have spells of severe dizziness
during exercise?   (No)   Yes

10. Do you experience unusual fatigue or shortness of breath
at rest or with mild exertion?   (No)   Yes

11. Have you had an attack of shortness of breath that came on
after you stopped exercising?   (No)   Yes

12. Have you been awakened at night by an attack of shortness
of breath?   (No)   Yes

13. Do you experience swelling or accumulation of fluid in or around
your ankles?   (No)   Yes

14. Do you often get the feeling that your heart is beating faster,
racing, or skipping beats, either at rest or during exercise?   (No)   Yes

15. Do you regularly get pains in your calves and lower legs during exercise which are not due to soreness or stiffness? (No) Yes

16. Has your doctor ever told you that you have a heart murmur? (No) Yes

Stage 3—Cardiac Risk Factors

17. Do you smoke cigarettes daily, or have you quit smoking within the past two years? No (Yes)

If yes, how many cigarettes per day do you smoke (or did you smoke in the past two years)? _10_ per day

18. Has your doctor ever told you that you have high blood pressure? No (Yes)

19. Has your father, mother, brother, or sister had a heart attack or suffered from cardiovascular disease before the age of 65? (No) Yes

If yes,

a) Was the relative male or female? _____

b) At what age did he or she have the stroke or heart attack? _____

c) Did this person die suddenly as a result of the stroke or heart attack? No Yes

20. Have you experienced menopause before the age of 45? No (Yes)

If yes, do you take hormone replacement medication? No (Yes)

If known, enter blood pressure and blood lipid values:

21. What is your systolic blood pressure? _136_ mmHg

22. What is your diastolic blood pressure? _78_ mmHg

23. What is your serum cholesterol level? _5.25_ (mmol/L) or mg/dL

24. What is your serum HDL level? _0.98_ (mmol/L) or mg/dL

25. What is your serum triglyceride level? _1.50_ (mmol/L) or mg/dL

Stage 4—Exercise Intentions

26. Does your job involve sitting for a large part of the day? No (Yes)

27. What are your current activity patterns?

a) Frequency: _Nil_ exercise sessions per week

b) Intensity: Sedentary Moderate Vigorous

c) History: <3 months 3–12 months >12 months

d) Duration: _____ minutes per session

28. What types of exercises do you do? _N/a_

29. Do you want to exercise at a moderate intensity (e.g., brisk walking) or at a vigorous intensity (e.g., jogging)? Moderate (Vigorous)

jogging in fun runs/circuit classes

HealthScreen Questionnaire

Name Jehan Åstrand   **Age** 74   **Gender** (M) F

Address _____

_____ **Phone** _____

Height 68.8 in (174.8 cm) **Mass** 160 lb (72.8 kg) **Date of test** _____

Profession retired engineer _____

Stage 1—Known Diseases (Medical Conditions)

1. List the medications you take on a regular basis.   none

2. Do you have diabetes?   No (Yes)

   a) If yes, please indicate if it is insulin-dependent diabetes mellitus (IDDM) or non–insulin-dependent diabetes mellitus (NIDDM).   IDDM (NIDDM)

   b) If IDDM, for how many years have you had IDDM?   _____ years

3. Have you had a stroke?   (No) Yes

4. Has your doctor ever said you have heart trouble?   (No) Yes

5. Do you take asthma medication?   (No) Yes

6. Are you or do you have reason to believe you may be pregnant?   (No) Yes

7. Is there any other physical reason that prevents you from participating in an exercise program (e.g., cancer; osteoporosis; severe arthritis; mental illness; thyroid, kidney, or liver disease)?   (No) Yes

Stage 2—Signs and Symptoms

8. Do you often have pains in your heart, chest, or surrounding areas, especially during exercise?   (No) Yes

9. Do you often feel faint or have spells of severe dizziness during exercise?   (No) Yes

10. Do you experience unusual fatigue or shortness of breath at rest or with mild exertion?   (No) Yes

11. Have you had an attack of shortness of breath that came on after you stopped exercising?   (No) Yes

12. Have you been awakened at night by an attack of shortness of breath?   (No) Yes

13. Do you experience swelling or accumulation of fluid in or around your ankles?   (No) Yes

14. Do you often get the feeling that your heart is beating faster, racing, or skipping beats, either at rest or during exercise?   (No) Yes

15. Do you regularly get pains in your calves and lower legs during exercise which are not due to soreness or stiffness? (No) Yes

16. Has your doctor ever told you that you have a heart murmur? (No) Yes

Stage 3—Cardiac Risk Factors

17. Do you smoke cigarettes daily, or have you quit smoking within the past two years? (No) Yes

    If yes, how many cigarettes per day do you smoke (or did you smoke in the past two years)? _____ per day

18. Has your doctor ever told you that you have high blood pressure? No (Yes)

19. Has your father, mother, brother, or sister had a heart attack or suffered from cardiovascular disease before the age of 65? (No) Yes

    If yes,

    a) Was the relative male or female? _____

    b) At what age did he or she have the stroke or heart attack? _____

    c) Did this person die suddenly as a result of the stroke or heart attack? No Yes

20. Have you experienced menopause before the age of 45? No Yes

    If yes, do you take hormone replacement medication? No Yes

If known, enter blood pressure and blood lipid values:

21. What is your systolic blood pressure? _155_ mmHg

22. What is your diastolic blood pressure? _98_ mmHg

23. What is your serum cholesterol level? _6.4_ (mmol/L) or mg/dL

24. What is your serum HDL level? _0.90_ (mmol/L) or mg/dL

25. What is your serum triglyceride level? _1.27_ (mmol/L) or mg/dL

Stage 4—Exercise Intentions

26. Does your job involve sitting for a large part of the day? No (Yes)

27. What are your current activity patterns?

    a) Frequency: _Nil_ exercise sessions per week

    b) Intensity: Sedentary Moderate Vigorous

    c) History: <3 months 3–12 months >12 months

    d) Duration: _____ minutes per session

28. What types of exercises do you do?

29. Do you want to exercise at a moderate intensity (e.g., brisk walking) or at a vigorous intensity (e.g., jogging)? (Moderate) Vigorous

HealthScreen Questionnaire

Name _Enoch Duke_   **Age** _22_   **Gender** (M)   F

Address _____

_____ **Phone** _____

Height _74.3 in (188.7 cm)_ **Mass** _175 lb (79.2 kg)_ **Date of test** _____

Profession _student_ _____

Stage 1—Known Diseases (Medical Conditions)

1. List the medications you take on a regular basis.   _none_

2. Do you have diabetes?   (No)   Yes

    a) If yes, please indicate if it is insulin-dependent diabetes mellitus (IDDM) or non–insulin-dependent diabetes mellitus (NIDDM).   IDDM   NIDDM

    b) If IDDM, for how many years have you had IDDM?   _____ years

3. Have you had a stroke?   (No)   Yes

4. Has your doctor ever said you have heart trouble?   (No)   Yes

5. Do you take asthma medication?   (No)   Yes

6. Are you or do you have reason to believe you may be pregnant?   (No)   Yes

7. Is there any other physical reason that prevents you from participating in an exercise program (e.g., cancer; osteoporosis; severe arthritis; mental illness; thyroid, kidney, or liver disease)?   (No)   Yes

Stage 2—Signs and Symptoms

8. Do you often have pains in your heart, chest, or surrounding areas, especially during exercise?   (No)   Yes

9. Do you often feel faint or have spells of severe dizziness during exercise?   (No)   Yes

10. Do you experience unusual fatigue or shortness of breath at rest or with mild exertion?   (No)   Yes

11. Have you had an attack of shortness of breath that came on after you stopped exercising?   (No)   Yes

12. Have you been awakened at night by an attack of shortness of breath?   (No)   Yes

13. Do you experience swelling or accumulation of fluid in or around your ankles?   (No)   Yes

14. Do you often get the feeling that your heart is beating faster, racing, or skipping beats, either at rest or during exercise?   (No)   Yes

15. Do you regularly get pains in your calves and lower legs during exercise which are not due to soreness or stiffness?   (No)   Yes

16. Has your doctor ever told you that you have a heart murmur?   (No)   Yes

Stage 3—Cardiac Risk Factors

17. Do you smoke cigarettes daily, or have you quit smoking within the past two years?   (No)   Yes

    If yes, how many cigarettes per day do you smoke (or did you smoke in the past two years)?   _____ per day

18. Has your doctor ever told you that you have high blood pressure?   (No)   Yes

19. Has your father, mother, brother, or sister had a heart attack or suffered from cardiovascular disease before the age of 65?   (No)   Yes

    If yes,

    a) Was the relative male or female?   _____

    b) At what age did he or she have the stroke or heart attack?   _____

    c) Did this person die suddenly as a result of the stroke or heart attack?   No   Yes

20. Have you experienced menopause before the age of 45?   No   Yes

    If yes, do you take hormone replacement medication?   No   Yes

If known, enter blood pressure and blood lipid values:

21. What is your systolic blood pressure?   _____mmHg

22. What is your diastolic blood pressure?   _____mmHg

23. What is your serum cholesterol level?   _____mmol/L or mg/dL

24. What is your serum HDL level?   _____mmol/L or mg/dL

25. What is your serum triglyceride level?   _____mmol/L or mg/dL

Stage 4—Exercise Intentions

26. Does your job involve sitting for a large part of the day?   No   (Yes)

27. What are your current activity patterns?
    a) Frequency: __2__ exercise sessions per week
    b) Intensity: Sedentary   Moderate   (Vigorous)
    c) History: <3 months (3–12 months) >12 months
    d) Duration: __30__ minutes per session

28. What types of exercises do you do? *weight lifting*

29. Do you want to exercise at a moderate intensity (e.g., brisk walking) or at a vigorous intensity (e.g., jogging)?   Moderate   (Vigorous)

HealthScreen Questionnaire

Name *Moira Lara*   **Age** *37*   **Gender**   M Ⓕ

Address _____

_____ **Phone** _____

Height *59 in (150.1 cm)* **Mass** *144 lb (65.1 kg)* **Date of test** _____

Profession *Lawyer* _____

Stage 1—Known Diseases (Medical Conditions)

1. List the medications you take on a regular basis.

2. Do you have diabetes?   Ⓝⓞ   Yes

   a) If yes, please indicate if it is insulin-dependent diabetes mellitus
   (IDDM) or non–insulin-dependent diabetes mellitus (NIDDM).   IDDM   NIDDM

   b) If IDDM, for how many years have you had IDDM?   _____ years

3. Have you had a stroke?   Ⓝⓞ   Yes

4. Has your doctor ever said you have heart trouble?   Ⓝⓞ   Yes

5. Do you take asthma medication?   Ⓝⓞ   Yes

6. Are you or do you have reason to believe you may be pregnant?   No   Ⓨⓔⓢ

7. Is there any other physical reason that prevents you
   from participating in an exercise program (e.g., cancer;
   osteoporosis; severe arthritis; mental illness; thyroid, kidney,
   or liver disease)?   Ⓝⓞ   Yes

Stage 2—Signs and Symptoms

8. Do you often have pains in your heart, chest, or surrounding
   areas, especially during exercise?   Ⓝⓞ   Yes

9. Do you often feel faint or have spells of severe dizziness
   during exercise?   Ⓝⓞ   Yes

10. Do you experience unusual fatigue or shortness of breath
    at rest or with mild exertion?   Ⓝⓞ   Yes

11. Have you had an attack of shortness of breath that came on
    after you stopped exercising?   Ⓝⓞ   Yes

12. Have you been awakened at night by an attack of shortness
    of breath?   Ⓝⓞ   Yes

13. Do you experience swelling or accumulation of fluid in or around
    your ankles?   Ⓝⓞ   Yes

14. Do you often get the feeling that your heart is beating faster,
    racing, or skipping beats, either at rest or during exercise?   Ⓝⓞ   Yes

15. Do you regularly get pains in your calves and lower legs during exercise which are not due to soreness or stiffness?   (No)   Yes

16. Has your doctor ever told you that you have a heart murmur?   (No)   Yes

Stage 3—Cardiac Risk Factors

17. Do you smoke cigarettes daily, or have you quit smoking within the past two years?   (No)   Yes

    If yes, how many cigarettes per day do you smoke (or did you smoke in the past two years)?   _____ per day

18. Has your doctor ever told you that you have high blood pressure?   (No)   Yes

19. Has your father, mother, brother, or sister had a heart attack or suffered from cardiovascular disease before the age of 65?   (No)   Yes

    If yes,

    a) Was the relative male or female?   _____

    b) At what age did he or she have the stroke or heart attack?   _____

    c) Did this person die suddenly as a result of the stroke or heart attack?   No   Yes

20. Have you experienced menopause before the age of 45?   (No)   Yes

    If yes, do you take hormone replacement medication?   No   Yes

If known, enter blood pressure and blood lipid values:

21. What is your systolic blood pressure?   _130_ mmHg

22. What is your diastolic blood pressure?   _68_ mmHg

23. What is your serum cholesterol level?   _−_ mmol/L or mg/dL

24. What is your serum HDL level?   _−_ mmol/L or mg/dL

25. What is your serum triglyceride level?   _−_ mmol/L or mg/dL

Stage 4—Exercise Intentions

26. Does your job involve sitting for a large part of the day?   No   (Yes)

27. What are your current activity patterns?

    a) Frequency: _2_ exercise sessions per week

    b) Intensity: Sedentary   (Moderate)   Vigorous

    c) History: (<3 months)   3–12 months   >12 months

    d) Duration: _20_ minutes per session

28. What types of exercises do you do?   *Walking*

29. Do you want to exercise at a moderate intensity (e.g., brisk walking) or at a vigorous intensity (e.g., jogging)?   (Moderate)   Vigorous

HealthScreen Questionnaire

Name <u>Magnus Gormley</u>   Age <u>47</u>   Gender (M) F

Address _____

_____ Phone _____

Height <u>65 in (165.4 cm)</u> Mass <u>179 lb (81.1 kg)</u> Date of test _____

Profession <u>biomechanist</u> _____

Stage 1—Known Diseases (Medical Conditions)

1. List the medications you take on a regular basis.   **none**

2. Do you have diabetes?   (No)   Yes

    a) If yes, please indicate if it is insulin-dependent diabetes mellitus
       (IDDM) or non–insulin-dependent diabetes mellitus (NIDDM).   IDDM NIDDM

    b) If IDDM, for how many years have you had IDDM?   _____ years

3. Have you had a stroke?   (No)   Yes

4. Has your doctor ever said you have heart trouble?   (No)   Yes

5. Do you take asthma medication?   (No)   Yes

6. Are you or do you have reason to believe you may be pregnant?   (No)   Yes

7. Is there any other physical reason that prevents you
    from participating in an exercise program (e.g., cancer;
    osteoporosis; severe arthritis; mental illness; thyroid, kidney,
    or liver disease)?   (No)   Yes

Stage 2—Signs and Symptoms

8. Do you often have pains in your heart, chest, or surrounding
    areas, especially during exercise?   (No)   Yes

9. Do you often feel faint or have spells of severe dizziness
    during exercise?   (No)   Yes

10. Do you experience unusual fatigue or shortness of breath
    at rest or with mild exertion?   No   (Yes)

11. Have you had an attack of shortness of breath that came on
    after you stopped exercising?   (No)   Yes

12. Have you been awakened at night by an attack of shortness
    of breath?   (No)   Yes

13. Do you experience swelling or accumulation of fluid in or around
    your ankles?   (No)   Yes

14. Do you often get the feeling that your heart is beating faster,
    racing, or skipping beats, either at rest or during exercise?   (No)   Yes

15. Do you regularly get pains in your calves and lower legs during exercise which are not due to soreness or stiffness?   (No)   Yes

16. Has your doctor ever told you that you have a heart murmur?   (No)   Yes

Stage 3—Cardiac Risk Factors

17. Do you smoke cigarettes daily, or have you quit smoking within the past two years?   No   (Yes)

    If yes, how many cigarettes per day do you smoke (or did you smoke in the past two years)?   **was: 25** per day
    I gave up last month

18. Has your doctor ever told you that you have high blood pressure?   (No)   Yes

19. Has your father, mother, brother, or sister had a heart attack or suffered from cardiovascular disease before the age of 65?   (No)   Yes

    If yes,

    a) Was the relative male or female?   _____

    b) At what age did he or she have the stroke or heart attack?   _____

    c) Did this person die suddenly as a result of the stroke or heart attack?   No   Yes

20. Have you experienced menopause before the age of 45?   No   Yes

    If yes, do you take hormone replacement medication?   No   Yes

If known, enter blood pressure and blood lipid values:

21. What is your systolic blood pressure?   **150** mmHg

22. What is your diastolic blood pressure?   **96** mmHg

23. What is your serum cholesterol level?   _____mmol/L or mg/dL

24. What is your serum HDL level?   _____mmol/L or mg/dL

25. What is your serum triglyceride level?   _____mmol/L or mg/dL

Stage 4—Exercise Intentions

26. Does your job involve sitting for a large part of the day?   No   (Yes)

27. What are your current activity patterns?

    a) Frequency: __nil_ exercise sessions per week

    b) Intensity: Sedentary   Moderate   Vigorous

    c) History: <3 months   3–12 months   >12 months

    d) Duration: _____minutes per session

28. What types of exercises do you do?   **nothing**

29. Do you want to exercise at a moderate intensity (e.g., brisk walking) or at a vigorous intensity (e.g., jogging)?   (Moderate)   Vigorous

screening judgments

▶ **Practice Case #1: Annabelle Mant**

1. Does this subject need a medical check-up and stress ECG before undertaking an exercise program? **No**

2. Does this subject need a medical doctor present during a maximal exercise test? **No**

3. Does this subject need a medical doctor present during a submaximal exercise test? **No**

Comments: Annabelle has no risk factors, is young, and only wants to engage in moderate exercise.

▶ **Practice Case #2: Karma Pope**

1. Does this subject need a medical check-up and stress ECG before undertaking an exercise program? **Yes**

2. Does this subject need a medical doctor present during a maximal exercise test? **Yes**

3. Does this subject need a medical doctor present during a submaximal exercise test? **Yes**

Comments: Karma has uncontrolled asthma (she takes asthma medication but still reports breathing difficulties).

▶ **Practice Case #3: Dougall Thompson**

1. Does this subject need a medical check-up and stress ECG before undertaking an exercise program? **No**

2. Does this subject need a medical doctor present during a maximal exercise test? **Yes**

3. Does this subject need a medical doctor present during a submaximal exercise test? **No**

Comments: Dougall has two risk factors (cholesterol and sedentarism) and is over 40. Because he only wants to exercise moderately, however, he does not need a check-up.

▶ **Practice Case #4: Alanna Etheridge**

1. Does this subject need a medical check-up and stress ECG before undertaking an exercise program? **Yes**

2. Does this subject need a medical doctor present during a maximal exercise test? **Yes**

3. Does this subject need a medical doctor present during a submaximal exercise test? **No**

Comments: Alanna has three cardiac risk factors: she smokes, is sedentary, and has a family history of cardiovascular disease. Although she is young, she wants to exercise vigorously.

▶ Practice Case #5: Vernon Ingleson

1. Does this subject need a medical check-up and stress ECG before undertaking an exercise program? **Yes**

2. Does this subject need a medical doctor present during a maximal exercise test? **Yes**

3. Does this subject need a medical doctor present during a submaximal exercise test? **No**

Comments: Vernon has four cardiac risk factors: age, high blood pressure, high cholesterol/low HDL, and sedentarism. He is also 71 years old and wants to do vigorous exercise.

▶ Practice Case #6: Sabine Andrews

1. Does this subject need a medical check-up and stress ECG before undertaking an exercise program? **Yes**

2. Does this subject need a medical doctor present during a maximal exercise test? **Yes**

3. Does this subject need a medical doctor present during a submaximal exercise test? **No**

Comments: Sabine has three cardiac risk factors: smoking, high cholesterol, and sedentarism. Although she experienced premature menopause, Sabine takes hormone replacement medication (Premarin), so she does not receive an additional cardiac risk factor.

▶ Practice Case #7: Jehan Åstrand

1. Does this subject need a medical check-up and stress ECG before undertaking an exercise program? **Yes**

2. Does this subject need a medical doctor present during a maximal exercise test? **Yes**

3. Does this subject need a medical doctor present during a submaximal exercise test? **Yes**

Comments: Jehan's diabetes counts as a known disease (he has NIDDM and is over 35 years old).

▶ **Practice Case #8: Enoch Duke**

1. Does this subject need a medical check-up and stress ECG before undertaking an exercise program? **No**

2. Does this subject need a medical doctor present during a maximal exercise test? **No**

3. Does this subject need a medical doctor present during a submaximal exercise test? **No**

Comments: Enoch has no known disease or signs and symptoms of disease but determining his cardiac risk factor status requires a judgment call. Enoch has no apparent cardiac risk factors, but he does not know his blood pressure and cholesterol values so you must insert population norms. If you use mean values for systolic and diastolic blood pressure and total cholesterol, Enoch will not receive any cardiac risk factors. If you assume Enoch is at low risk, however, he will receive a cardiac risk factor for total cholesterol or low HDL, but the screening judgment remains the same.

▶ **Practice Case #9 : Moira Lara**

1. Does this subject need a medical check-up and stress ECG before undertaking an exercise program? **Yes**

2. Does this subject need a medical doctor present during a maximal exercise test? **Yes**

3. Does this subject need a medical doctor present during a submaximal exercise test? **Yes**

Comments: Moira indicates that she is (or might be) pregnant on her questionnaire, so she is treated as if she has a known disease.

▶ **Practice Case #10: Magnus Gormley**

1. Does this subject need a medical check-up and stress ECG before undertaking an exercise program? **Yes**

2. Does this subject need a medical doctor present during a maximal exercise test? **Yes**

3. Does this subject need a medical doctor present during a submaximal exercise test? **Yes**

Comments: Magnus indicates that he has experienced "unusual fatigue or shortness of breath at rest or with mild exertion," which can be a symptom of underlying cardiopulmonary disease.

a pharmacopoeia

There are many reasons why it is useful for the person conducting pre-exercise screening to know a little about the drugs people are taking. It helps them to put together a picture of the health status of the person being screened. Conditions such as heart disease, severe asthma, metabolic disease, and arthritis may mean that the person being screened needs a medical check-up before exercise.

Some people are not always aware of the nature and purpose of the drugs they are taking—they simply "follow doctor's orders." There are also some drugs that may affect pre-exercise screening results. For example, oral contraceptives may produce unusual blood lipid values.

A pharmacopoeia is a list of drugs and their actions. Below is a list of some drugs commonly used in Australia and some of their common actions. This list is intended as a guide only. Many drugs have a number of uses, and if there is any doubt the sports health care provider or EP should consult a pharmacist or medical doctor.

▶ A

Actifed Contains pseudoephedrine, which is used as a decongestant and antihistamine.

Actrapid Rapidly acting insulin injection. Peaks two to five hours after injection.

Adalat Calcium-channel blocker used for angina.

Aldactone Diuretic.

Aldomet Antihypertensive agent, which reduces both supine and standing blood pressure.

Alupent Bronchodilator used for asthma.

Amoxil Antibiotic.

Ampicyn Semisynthetic penicillin.

Anginine Vasodilator used to relieve angina pectoris.

Apresoline Antihypertensive agent that works by directly relaxing arterioles.

Aprinox Diuretic.

Aspirin Analgesic that can also be used as an anticoagulant.

Atrovent Anticholinergic bronchodilator used for asthma.

▶ **B**

Bactrim Antibacterial drug used especially for respiratory and urinary infections.

Beconase Inhaled corticosteroid used for allergic rhinitis.

Becotide Inhaled anti-inflammatory agent used in long-term asthma management.

Benemid Used to treat gout. It works by inhibiting renal reabsorption of urates.

Berotec Beta-agonist inhalant used as bronchodilator to treat asthma.

Betaloc A beta-adrenergic blocker used to treat high blood pressure.

Betaplex Vitamin supplement.

Bricanyl Beta-agonist used as bronchodilator for acute relief of bronchial asthma.

Brufen Common nonsteroidal anti-inflammatory drug (NSAID). Often used for arthritis.

▶ **C**

Calvita Vitamin and calcium supplement.

Capoten An antihypertensive that is an ACE (angiotensin-converting enzyme) inhibitor.

Cartia Aspirin. Often used as an anticoagulant and antithrombosis drug.

Celestone Corticosteroid that can be taken orally or applied as a cream. Used mainly for skin disorders.

Chlotride Diuretic.

Codeine Analgesic. Codeine is metabolized in the liver to form morphine.

Codral Analgesic and antipyretic. Used to treat headaches and the symptoms of flu.

Codral Aspirin and pseudoephedrine. Used as a decongestant and antihistamine.

Cordilox A calcium-channel blocker that relaxes cardiac and vascular smooth muscle and lowers blood pressure.

▶ **D**

De-Nol Heals gastric ulcers.

Deca-Durabolin Anabolic steroid used in acute renal failure and anemia.

Diabex Oral hypoglycemic used to treat non-insulin-dependent diabetes mellitus (NIDDM).

Diamicron Oral hypoglycemic used in the treatment of NIDDM.

Diazepam Sedative and anti-anxiety drug. Valium and Ducene contain diazepam.

Dilantin Anticonvulsant drug used in the treatment of epilepsy.

Dindevan Anticoagulant that prevents the formation of clotting factors.

Ducene Sedative and anti-anxiety drug.

Durabolin Anabolic steroid used in acute renal failure and anemia.

Dyazide Diuretic.

Dymadon Paracetamol, an analgesic and antipyretic.

► **E**

Ecotrin Aspirin tablets designed for people who do not tolerate aspirin well.

Enduron Diuretic.

Epilim Anticonvulsant used in the treatment of epilepsy.

Ergodryl Vasoconstricts cranial blood vessels. Used in the treatment of migraines.

Ergomatine Vasoconstricts cranial blood vessels. Used in the treatment of migraines.

Estigyn Estrogen used to treat amenorrhea and dysmenorrhea.

Euglucon Oral hypoglycemic used in the treatment of NIDDM.

► **F**

Feritard Iron supplement.

► **G**

Gaviscon Antacid used in the treatment of ulcers.

Gerovit Vitamin supplement often used for older subjects.

► **H**

Hormone replacement therapy (HRT) Used in post-menopausal women to treat symptoms such as hot flushes.

Hydrocortisone Topical corticosteroid for skin rashes.

Hygroton Diuretic.

► **I**

Ibuprofen Common NSAID. Often used in treatment of arthritis.

Imiprin Tricyclic antidepressant.

Inderal Beta-adrenergic blocker used to reduce blood pressure.

Indocid NSAID that inhibits prostaglandin synthesis. Often used in treatment of arthritis.

Insulin Used with diabetics to help glucose transport into the cells.

Intal Sodium chromoglycate. Inhibits the release of mediators of allergic response. Used for bronchial asthma.

Isomil Soy protein milk substitute used for patients with lactose intolerance.

Isoptin A calcium-channel blocker that relaxes cardiac and vascular smooth muscle and lowers blood pressure. It is also used to reduce arrhythmia.

Isordil Vasodilator that affects peripheral vasculature and reduces preload on the heart.

► **L**

Lanoxin Digoxin. Increases force of heart contractions and increases cardiac output.

Largactil Major tranquilizer used with mental patients.

Lasix Diuretic.

Lente Slower-acting insulin injection. Peaks 7 to 15 hours after injection.

Librium Sedative and anti-anxiety drug also used as a muscle relaxant.

Lithium Antidepressant.

Lomotil Drug used to treat diarrhea.

Lopresor Beta-adrenergic blocker used to reduce blood pressure.

► **M**

Midamor Diuretic.

Minipress Vasodilator used to reduce blood pressure.

Minirin Antidiuretic used to treat diabetes insipidus.

Mogadon Sedative.

Moxacin Semisynthetic penicillin. Antibiotic.

Murelax Anti-anxiety drug.

Mylanta Antacid and antiflatulent used in the treatment of ulcers.

Mysteclin Broad spectrum antibiotic.

► **N**

Naprosyn NSAID used in treatment of arthritis and dysmenorrhea.

Natrilix Diuretic.

Nembutal Sedative and hypnotic used for insomnia and pre-op.

Nordette A contraceptive pill.

Nuelin Theophylline. Relaxes smooth bronchial muscle. Asthma drug.

► **O**

Ogen Estrogen used in hormone replacement therapy.

Oroxine Thyroid replacement hormone.

Orthoxicol Used to treat common cold or flu.

Orudis NSAID used in treatment of arthritis.

► **P**

Panadol Paracetamol, an analgesic and antipyretic.

Panamax Paracetamol, an analgesic and antipyretic.

Paracetamol Analgesic and antipyretic.

Paroven Decreases capillary fragility and permeability and increases venous return. Used for treating varicose veins and edema.

Periactin Serotonin and histamine antagonist. Anti-allergy drug.

Plaquenil Used to treat lupus erythematosus and severe arthritis.

Polaramine Antihistamine and antitussive.

Ponderax Fenfluramine, an appetite suppressant.

Prednisolone Corticosteroid used in the management of asthma.

Premarin Estrogen used in hormone replacement therapy. It is also used to strengthen capillary walls and enhance coagulation.

Prothiaden Tricyclic antidepressant.

Provera Used to treat endometrial cancer and endometriosis. Has also been used—controversially—as a contraceptive.

Pulmacort Inhaled anti-inflammatory agent used in long-term asthma management.

▶ **Q**

Questran A hypolipidemic drug used to lower cholesterol.

Quinidine Anti-arrhythmic drug.

Quinine Used to treat malaria. Also used as a muscle relaxant to treat cramps.

▶ **R**

Ranitidine Histamine antagonist used to treat ulcers.

Respolin Salbutamol tablets for relief of bronchospasm. Asthma drug.

Ritalin Amphetamine-like drug often used to treat hyperactivity in children, for whom it may have the opposite effect.

Rohypnol Sedative and hypnotic.

Rynacrom Sodium chromoglycate. Nasal spray for allergic rhinitis.

▶ **S**

Salazopyrin Used to treat inflammation of the colon (colitis).

Sandomigran Used to treat migraines.

Senokot Laxative used to treat constipation.

Seprin Antibacterial drug used especially for respiratory and urinary infections.

Serenace Psychotropic drug used to control paranoia and mania.

Sinutab Used to relieve common cold and flu.

Slow-K Treatment for hypokalemia, which often accompanies the use of diuretics.

Spironolactone Generic name for a potassium-sparing diuretic.

Spirotone Potassium-sparing diuretic.

Stelazine Used to control excessive anxiety and tension. Also used as an antinausea drug.

Stemetil Antinausea drug.

Stilbesterol Synthetic estrogen used to treat menstrual dysfunction.

Sudafed Contains pseudoephedrine, which is used as a decongestant and antihistamine.

▶ **T**

Tegretol Depresses synaptic transmission in the central nervous system. Used as an anticonvulsant in the treatment of epilepsy.

Tenormin A beta-adrenergic blocker used to treat high blood pressure.

Tetrex Broad spectrum antibiotic.

Theo-Dur Theophylline. Relaxes smooth bronchial muscle. Asthma drug.

Thyroxine Generic name for thyroid replacement hormone.

Timoptol Reduces intra-ocular pressure, which often occurs with glaucoma.

Trasicor Beta-adrenergic blocker used to reduce blood pressure.

▶ **U**

Ultralente Very slow-acting insulin injection. Peaks 18 to 24 hours after injection.

▶ V

Valium Sedative and anti-anxiety drug.

Ventolin Inhalant. A selective beta-agonist that dilates the airways. Asthma drug.

Verapamil A calcium-channel blocker that relaxes cardiac and vascular smooth muscle and lowers blood pressure.

Vibra-Tabs Broad spectrum antibiotic.

Visken Beta-adrenergic blocker used to reduce blood pressure.

Voltaren NSAID used to treat rheumatism and arthritis.

▶ Z

Zantac Histamine antagonist used to treat ulcers.

Zyloprim Used to treat gout. It inhibits an enzyme involved in the formation of uric acid.

bibliography

American College of Sports Medicine. 1975. *Guidelines for graded exercise testing and exercise prescription*. Philadelphia: Lea and Febiger.

———. 1980. *Guidelines for graded exercise testing and exercise prescription*. 2d ed. Philadelphia: Lea and Febiger.

———. 1986. *Guidelines for graded exercise testing and exercise prescription*. 3d ed. Philadelphia: Lea and Febiger.

———. 1991. *Guidelines for graded exercise testing and exercise prescription*. 4th ed. Philadelphia: Lea and Febiger.

———. 1995. *Guidelines for graded exercise testing and exercise prescription*. 5th ed. Baltimore: Williams and Wilkins.

Australian Institute of Health and Welfare. 1996. *Australia's health*. Canberra: Australian Government Printing Service.

Blair, S.N., Kampert, J.B., Kohl, H.W., Barlow, C.E., Macera, C.A., Paffenbarger, R.S., and Gibbons, L.W. 1996. Influences of cardiorespiratory fitness and other precursors on cardiovascular disease and all-cause mortality in men and women. *Journal of the American Medical Association* 276 (3):205-210.

Bowes, D. 1998. *The ACSM 1995 pre-exercise screening system: Who will be excluded?* Unpublished BSpSc (Hon) thesis, University of New South Wales.

Department of the Arts, Sport, the Environment and Territories (DASET). 1992. *Pilot survey of the fitness of Australians*. Canberra: Australian Government Printing Service.

Gilman, A.G., Rall, T.W., Nies, A.S., and Taylor, P., eds. 1991. *Goodman and Gilman's the pharmacological basis of therapeutics*. 8th ed. New York: Pergamon Press.

Gore, C.J., Owen, N., Dauman, A., and Booth, M. 1993. Methods of the pilot survey of the fitness of Australians. *Australian Journal of Science and Medicine in Sport* 25 (3):80-83.

Haskell, W.L. 1981. Cardiovascular complications during medically supervised exercise training. In *Physical conditioning and cardiovascular rehabilitation*, ed. L.S. Cohen, M.B. Mock, and I. Ringqvist, 159-167. New York: Wiley.

Herbert, D.L. 1995. More exercise testing litigation. *Exercise Standards and Malpractice Reporter* 9:30.

———. 1996. More exercise testing litigation. *Exercise Standards and Malpractice Reporter* 10:23-26.

Kannel, W.B. 1995. Epidemiologic insights into atherosclerotic cardiovascular disease—from the Framingham study. In *Heart disease and rehabilitation*, ed. M.L. Pollock and D.H. Schmidt, 3-16. Champaign, IL: Human Kinetics.

Knight, J.A., Laubach, C.A., Butcher, R.J., and Menapace, F.J. 1995. Supervision of clinical exercise testing by exercise physiologists. *American Journal of Cardiology* 75:390-391.

Kohl, H.W., Gibbons, L.W., Gordon, N.F., and Blair, S.N. 1990. An empirical evaluation of the ACSM guidelines for exercise testing. *Medicine and Science in Sports and Exercise* 22:533-539.

National Center for Health Statistics. 1994. *National health and nutrition examination survey (NHANES III), 1988-1994.* Hyattsville, MD: Public Health Service.

National Heart Foundation. 1995. *Heart and stroke facts.* Canberra: Australian Government Printing Service.

Neaton, J.D., and Wentworth, D. 1992. Serum cholesterol, blood pressure, cigarette smoking, and death from coronary heart disease. *Archives of Internal Medicine* 152:56-64.

Norton, K.I., Olds, T.S., Ly, S.V., and Gore, C.J. 1996. Exclusion rates using ACSM's pre-exercise screening procedures. *Medicine and Science in Sports and Exercise* 28 (5):S186.

Norton, K.I., Olds, T.S., Ly, S.V., Gore, C.J., and Bowes, D.J. 1998. Applying the SMA pre-exercise screening guidelines: Who will be excluded? *Journal of Science and Medicine in Sport* 1 (1):38-51.

Powell, K.E., Thompson, P.D., Caspersen, C.J., and Kendrick, J.S. 1987. Physical activity and the incidence of coronary heart disease. In *Annual review of public health*, ed. L. Breslow, J.E. Fielding, and L.B. Lave, 253-287. Palo Alto, CA: Annual Reviews, Inc.

Shephard, R.J. 1988. Par-Q, Canadian Home Fitness Test and exercise screening alternatives. *Sports Medicine* 5:193-201.

Shephard, R.J. 1991. Safety of exercise testing—the role of the paramedical specialist. *Clinical Journal of Sports Medicine* 1:8-11.

Siscovick, D.S., Weiss, N.S., Fletcher, R.H., and Lasky, T. 1984. The incidence of primary cardiac arrest during vigorous exercise. *New England Journal of Medicine* 311:874-877.

Siscovick, D.S. 1990. Risks of exercising: Sudden cardiac death and injuries. In *Exercise, fitness, and health*, ed. C. Bouchard, R. Shephard, T. Stephens, J. Sutton, and B. McPherson, 707-713. Champaign, IL: Human Kinetics.

Thompson, P.D. 1988. The safety of exercise testing and participation. In *Resource manual for guidelines for exercise testing and prescription*, ed. American College of Sports Medicine, 273-277. Philadelphia: Lea and Febiger.

———. 1993. Athletes, athletics, and sudden cardiac death. *Medicine and Science in Sports and Exercise* 25:983-988.

Thompson, P.D., and Fahrenbach, M.C. 1994. Risks of exercising: Cardiovascular including sudden cardiac death. In *Physical activity, fitness, and health*, ed. C. Bouchard, R. Shephard, T. Stephens, J. Sutton, and B. McPherson, 1019-1028. Champaign, IL: Human Kinetics.

Thompson, P.D., Funk, E.J., Carleton, R.A., and Sturner, W.Q. 1982. Incidence of death during jogging in Rhode Island from 1975 to 1980. *Journal of the American Medical Association* 247:2535-2538.

U.S. Department of Agriculture. 1994. Food consumption and expenditures, 1960-1993. *Statistical Bulletin* 915.

U.S. Department of Health and Human Services. 1996. *Physical activity and health: A report of the Surgeon General.* Atlanta, GA: U.S. Department of Health and Human Services, Centers for Disease Control and Prevention, National Center for Chronic Disease Prevention and Health Promotion, 111.

van Camp, S.P., and Peterson, R.A. 1986. Cardiovascular complications of outpatient cardiac rehabilitation programs. *Journal of the American Medical Association* 256:1160-1163.

Vuori, I. 1984. The cardiovascular risks of physical activity. *Acta Medica Scandinavica*, Suppl. 711:204-214.

Vuori, I., Suurnakki, L., and Suurnakki, T. 1982. Risk of sudden cardiovascular death (SCVD) in exercise. *Medicine and Science in Sports and Exercise* 14:114-115.

about the authors

Tim Olds, PhD, is a senior lecturer in the School of Physical Education, Exercise, and Sport Studies at the University of South Australia. Dr. Olds is the coeditor of *Anthropemetrica: A Textbook of Body Measurement for Sports and Health Courses* and cocreator of *HealthScreen* software, a pre-exercise screening tool. His research interests include mathematical modeling of sports performance, body composition, and anthropometry.

Kevin Norton, PhD, is an associate professor in the School of Physical Education, Exercise, and Sport Studies at the University of South Australia. Dr. Norton is the coeditor of *Anthropemetrica: A Textbook of Body Measurement for Sports and Health Courses* and cocreator of *HealthScreen* software, a pre-exercise screening tool. His research focuses on areas such as elite sports performance, respiratory function during exercise, and anthropometry. Dr. Norton has also worked full-time and as a consultant in the fitness industry for more than two decades.

Other Distance Education Courses

Advanced Flexibility for Fitness Professionals

1999 • Includes *Science of Flexibility*, 392 pp textbook; *Teaching Flexibility*, 51-minute video; and Self-Study Guide • Item CHKP0318 • ISBN 0-7360-0318-5
PAL Version: Item CHKP0319 • ISBN 0-7360-0319-3
Please call for CEU and price information

This course provides fitness specialists with a comprehensive understanding of the science of flexibility, increases their knowledge of specific flexibility exercises, and helps them correctly prescribe flexibility exercises for various populations and health conditions.

Assessing Body Composition

1999 • 78 pp Self-Study Guide and Body Composition Kit containing 17-minute video, skinfold calipers, measuring tape, and software
Item CHKP0145 • ISBN 0-7360-0145-X
$99.00 ($129.95 Canadian)
PAL Version: CHKP0179 • ISBN 0-7360-0179-4
£95.50 Europe ($141.00 Aus, $236.50 NZ)
Approved for 1.0 NSCA CEUs, 10 AEA CECs, and 2.5 AKTA CEUs

This concise, practical course will teach you how to more accurately assess body composition using skinfold calipers and software to calculate percent body fat, lean muscle mass, and much more.

Other Products

LifeSize

Dr. Tim Olds and Dr. Kevin Norton • University of South Australia
CD-ROM with approx. 56 pp user manual
1999 • LifeSize Agency Edition • Windows disk: Item MUSA0074 • Mac disk: Item MUSA0075 CD-ROM: Item MUSA0248 • $195.00 ($292.50 Cdn, £188.00 UK, $351.00 Aus, $466.50 NZ)
1999 • LifeSize Personal Edition • Windows disk: Item MUSA0076 • Mac disk: Item MUSA0077 CD-ROM: Item MUSA0247 • $49.00 ($73.50 Cdn, £47.00 UK, $88.50 Aus, $117.00 NZ)

Expand your body composition knowledge and skills with *LifeSize* software. This software program will first teach you and your students the exciting dimensions of anthropometry and will then make it easy for you to use anthropometry in class projects and research programs.

Health Fitness Instructor's Handbook (Third Edition)

Edward T. Howley, PhD, and B. Don Franks, PhD
1997 • Hardback • 552 pp • Item BHOW0958 • ISBN 0-87322-958-4
$45.00 ($67.50 Cdn, £37.00 UK, $81.00 Aus, $107.50 NZ)

Setting a new standard for texts on fitness testing and prescription, *Health Fitness Instructor's Handbook* is an indispensable reference for every health fitness instructor and exercise scientist.

To request more information including CEU availability or to order, U.S. customers call 1-800-747-4457, e-mail us at humank@hkusa.com, or visit our website at www.humankinetics.com. Persons outside the U.S. can contact us via our website or use the appropriate telephone number, postal address, or e-mail address shown in the front of this book.

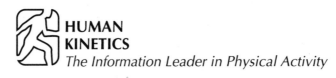

HUMAN KINETICS
The Information Leader in Physical Activity